**W9-BSJ-109**

"If you give yourself over wholeheartedly to what is being offered in this book, it could make an enormous difference in your life and health in important ways too numerous to count. The authors are committed practitioners of mindfulness and their mindfulness-based cancer recovery program, firmly rooted in research findings, radiates an authenticity that you can readily feel, and that will grow with time."

—Jon Kabat-Zinn, Ph.D., professor of medicine emeritus at University of Massachusetts Medical School

"*Mindfulness-Based Cancer Recovery* is a thoughtful, clear, and useful guide to living with cancer and cancer treatment, written by leading experts in the field. It distills Buddhist tradition into a series of practical exercises that can help you spend more of your time in the calm eye of the hurricane that is cancer."

—David Spiegel, MD, Willson Professor and associate chair of psychiatry and behavioral sciences at Stanford University School of Medicine

"Linda Carlson and Michael Speca have masterfully written a clear, insightful, and comprehensive book on coping with cancer. They beautifully weave together clinical wisdom, deep, personal mindfulness practice, and scientific rigor in their easily accessible book. I believe the wealth of ideas and practices in this book will be of benefit to those with cancer, offering a path toward greater ease, joy, health, and freedom both during treatment and beyond."

—Shauna L. Shapiro, associate professor at Santa Clara University and coauthor of *The Art and Science of Mindfulness*

"Linda Carlson and Michael Speca have cowritten this wise and practical guidebook, a generous offering to cancer patients and their allies. Those who find their way to it will certainly be blessed by their clear vision and deep experience."

—Sharon Salzberg, author of *Real Happiness*

MINDFULNESS-BASED
CANCER RECOVERY

A
Step-by-Step
MBSR Approach
to Help You
Cope with
Treatment &
Reclaim Your
Life

LINDA E. CARLSON, PH.D., R.PSYCH.
MICHAEL SPECA, PSY.D., R.PSYCH.

NEW HARBINGER PUBLICATIONS, INC.

Publisher's Note

Adapted from FULL CATASTROPHE LIVING by Jon Kabat-Zinn, copyright © 1990 by Jon Kabat-Zinn. Used by permission of Dell Publishing, a division of Random House, Inc.

"Love after Love" from COLLECTED POEMS 1948-1984 by Derek Walcott. Copyright © 1986 by Derek Walcott. Reprinted by permission of Farrar, Straus and Giroux, LLC.

"Seas" from THE SELECTED WRITINGS OF JUAN RAMON JIMENEZ by Juan Ramon Jimenez, translated by H.R. Hays. Copyright © 1957 by Juan Ramon Jimenez. Copyright renewed 1985 by Farrar, Straus and Giroux, LLC. Reprinted by permission of Farrar, Straus and Giroux, LLC.

"The Summer Day" from NEW AND SELECTED POEMS, VOLUME ONE by Mary Oliver. Copyright © 2004 by Mary Oliver. Reprinted by permission of Beacon Press, Boston.

"Wild Geese" from DREAM WORK by Mary Oliver. Copyright © 1994 by Mary Oliver. Reprinted by permission of Atlantic Monthly Press.

Insight Meditation: A Step-by-Step Course on How to Meditate by Sharon Salzberg and Joseph Goldstein. Copyright © 2002 Sharon Salzberg and Joseph Goldstein. All rights reserved. Used with permission from Sounds True, Inc., Boulder, Co, www.SoundsTrue.com.

"The Guest House" by Rumi, translated by Coleman Barks. All rights reserved. Reprinted with permission from Coleman Barks

"Love after Love" from COLLECTED POEMS 1948-1984 by Derek Walcott. Copyright © 1986 by Derek Walcott. Reprinted by permission of Farrar, Straus and Giroux, LLC.

"Seas" from THE SELECTED WRITINGS OF JUAN RAMON JIMENEZ by Juan Ramon Jimenez, translated by H.R. Hays. Copyright © 1957 by Juan Ramon Jimenez. Copyright renewed 1985 by Farrar, Straus and Giroux, LLC. Reprinted by permission of Farrar, Straus and Giroux, LLC.

"The Wanting Creature" from KABIR: ECSTATIC POEMS by Robert Bly. Copyright © 2004 by Robert Bly. Reprinted by permission of Beacon Press, Boston.

"My life is not this steeply sloping hour..." from SELECTED POEMS OF RAINER MARIA RILKE, translated by Robert Bly. Copyright 1981 ©. Reprinted by permission of HarperCollins Publishers.

Copyright © 2010 by Linda E. Carlson and Michael Speca
New Harbinger Publications, Inc.
5674 Shattuck Avenue
Oakland, CA 94609
www.newharbinger.com

All Rights Reserved
Printed in the United States of America
Distributed in Canada by Raincoast Books
Acquired by Tesilya Hanauer; Cover design by Amy Shoup; Edited by Nelda Street

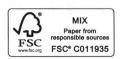

MIX
Paper from
responsible sources
FSC® C011935

Library of Congress Cataloging-in-Publication Data

Carlson, Linda E.

Mindfulness-based cancer recovery : a step-by-step MBSR approach to help you cope with treatment and reclaim your life / Linda E. Carlson and Michael P. Speca ; foreword by Zindel Segal.

  p. cm.

Includes bibliographical references.

  ISBN 978-1-57224-887-8 (pbk.) -- ISBN 978-1-57224-888-5 (pdf ebook)

  1. Cancer--Patients--Rehabilitation. 2. Cancer--Treatment--Psychological aspects. 3. Mindfulness-based cognitive therapy. 4. Stress (Psychology) 5. Stress management. 6. Relaxation. I. Speca, Michael P. II. Title.

RC262.C299 2010

616.99'406--dc22

                    2010043970

20 19 18

10 9 8 7 6 5 4

This book is dedicated to all the people who have shared their lives with us through participation in the mindfulness groups we have led over the past thirteen years. Their stories and bravery in the face of cancer continue to inspire us.

Contents

PART I
Setting the Stage

  ~ Outline of This Book ~ The Cancer Experience
  ~ What Is Mindfulness? ~ Roots of Mindfulness
  ~ Development of MBCR ~ Is Mindfulness for You?

  ~ The Stress Response ~ The Effects of Prolonged Stress
  ~ Recognizing Your Stress Symptoms ~ Where Does
Stress Come From? ~ Stress and the Mind-Body Connection
  ~ Mindfulness and Stress ~ Stress and Cancer ~ Coping
with Stress

PART II
The MBCR Program

PART III

Symptom Management and Everyday Mindfulness

Acknowledgments

We are pleased to be able to share the MBCR program with a wide audience, and have many parties to thank for making it possible to offer this book. In terms of academic support, Linda holds the Enbridge Research Chair in Psychosocial Oncology, cofunded by the Canadian Cancer Society Alberta/NWT Division and the Alberta Cancer Foundation. She also holds an Alberta Heritage Foundation for Medical Research Health Scholar Award. These awards provide protected time for research activities, which has made it possible to conduct the research behind this book.

Our professional colleagues in the Psychosocial Resources Department at the Tom Baker Cancer Centre, Alberta Health Services Cancer Care in Calgary, Alberta, Canada, have been supportive throughout the development of this program. Special thanks to our department head Barry Bultz, and all departmental counselors and researchers. Shirley McMillan, Maureen Angen, and Eileen Goodey have facilitated the MBCR program and contributed to its development. Their support and input have been essential to its ongoing success.

For our own practice of meditation and yoga, thanks go to the Insight Meditation Society, Sharon Salzberg, Jack Kornfield, and Thich Nhat Hanh. While studying dance at SUNY, Brockport, Michael was introduced to yoga by Peentz Dubble, who is now an accomplished Iyengar yoga instructor in the Boston area, and he began sitting meditation practice with friends from the nearby Rochester Zen Center, founded by Philip Kapleau Roshi. Jon Kabat-Zinn has been a friend, colleague, and mentor, as well as a primary inspiration for the MBCR program. Saki Santorelli, current director of the Center for Mindfulness, has been inspiring and supportive. Linda thanks her colleagues at the Mind and Life Institute for providing exposure to an international array of meditation researchers and practitioners; special thanks to Adam Engle, Richie Davidson, Joan Halifax, David Meyer, Al Kaszniak, Evan Thompson, John Dunne, and Zindel Segal.

Michael would like to express his gratitude for the late Cynthia Novack and the late Richard Bull, dance choreographers and teachers who demonstrated the vital role of awareness in the grand improvisation that is life, and to Susan Foster for introducing him to mind-body studies.

Our students have been instrumental in helping conduct and conceptualize our research on mindfulness; special thanks go to Sheila Garland, Laura Labelle, Michael Mackenzie, Katie Birnie, Kristin Zernicke, Sarah Cook, Marion Hutchins, and Laura Lansdell. Over the years several research assistants have also provided essential contributions to these projects: Barbara Pickering, Linette Lawlor-Savage, Joshua Lounsberry, Beth DeBruyn, and Andrea Berenbaum. Special acknowledgment goes to Andrea Berenbaum, who through superior artistic and computer skills created the illustrations seen throughout this book.

Personal thanks are also due to those in our private lives who took over duties at home or family responsibilities to allow us the time to work on this book. Linda thanks Joal Borggard for his love, support, and understanding, and her daughter Nova for being a natural and joyful practitioner of beginner's mind. The new arrival of son Vardin coincides with the birth of this book, and it will be enjoyable to see both grow as they are introduced to the world. She also thanks her parents Lorne and Shirley Carlson for all their support and encouragement over the years.

Michael thanks his wife and best friend Nancy (Ford) Speca for her love and for encouraging him to be his best self, his mother Joan (Slaven) Speca for her love and support, and father Annibale (William) Speca who faced cancer with grace and courage.

Foreword

The experience of cancer is rarely defined by discrete events as much as it is by a process of linkage among the specific stages that mark one's progress through receiving a diagnosis, deciding on treatment, completing treatment, recovering functional capacity, and then living with an ever-present vigilance for signs of its return or durable remission. How can we respond to these challenges that, even though unbidden, nevertheless require our engagement? Can we harness the power residing in the mind to develop a healing perspective and apply it in those very moments when we become lost in thoughts, worries, or disturbing scenarios about a limited future? Mindfulness-based cancer recovery (MBCR), the program developed by Linda Carlson and Michael Speca in 1995 and clearly described in this accessible and pragmatic workbook, provides patients with the opportunity to find their own answers to these inevitable questions along with concrete skills for embedding them into everyday life.

The eight-week MBCR program is characterized by the clinical application of meditative practices that are designed to help patients develop a particular form of awareness, known as mindfulness. The origins of mindfulness can be traced to the wisdom traditions of Asia, where it has been taught for over 2,500 years. MBCR is part of a recent trend that has seen these practices adapted for use in Western medicine. This turns out to be a productive union, since the standard forms of cancer care such as medication, surgery, chemotherapy, and radiation therapy are rarely sufficient to meet patients' ongoing needs. In going through the program, patients first learn about the differences between responding to events automatically and doing so with an awareness of what is going on in the body and the mind. The simple yet powerful role of attention in anchoring in the present moment a mind that is carried away by endless rumination, catastrophizing, or angst turns out to be one of the most important supports that people can naturally call on. Once this ability is more firmly in place, the workbook moves through the myriad of difficulties brought on by the experience of cancer to suggest ways mindfulness can inform a compassionate and skillful means of caring for oneself.

The effectiveness of MBCR stems from its focus on the whole person and not just the cancer diagnosis. Presented within a logical modular structure, chapters devoted to coping with the side effects of somatic treatments such as hair loss, fatigue, and pain sit alongside accessible descriptions of how mindfulness can help in managing the daily challenges of stress, isolation, and changes in self-perception. The thread running throughout this work is that mindful awareness is the best starting point for addressing one's needs, even if the outcome of doing so is not always guaranteed. Illustrations of how mindfulness can be practiced—both formally and informally, while sitting still or in motion, for long periods or only briefly—reinforce the flexibility inherent in this approach and reduce barriers to its implementation.

The first line in chapter 1 of this book poses the question "How can mindfulness help you cope with cancer?" In Mindfulness-Based Cancer Recovery, readers will find an answer that is both tangible and evolving. In illuminating the working edge between what is needed in the short term and what is possible in the long term, Carlson and Speca have provided a valuable resource for compassionate and clear-sighted care through one of the most difficult health journeys we may ever find ourselves embarking upon.

—Zindel V. Segal, Ph.D.
　Cameron Wilson Chair in Depression Studies
　Professor of Psychiatry, University of Toronto

PART I

Setting the Stage

CHAPTER 1

Mindfulness and Cancer

How can mindfulness help you cope with cancer? Answering this question forms the basis of this book. If you are reading these pages, you have likely encountered some of the rites of passage people being treated for cancer and their families and friends experience, including the shock of the initial diagnosis and whirlwind of tests and treatments; waiting rooms; exams; confusing medical speak; and fears of pain, suffering, and loss. In addition, you may hold some ideas or simply be curious to learn more about how mindfulness or meditation could help in the face of cancer. We don't offer you mindfulness as a cure for your disease. Rather, it holds the possibility of vastly enriching your life, helping you cope with symptoms and side effects, and improving the quality of your days. Mindfulness may also enhance your immune system's performance and help reduce harmful levels of stress hormones in your body, changes that can only be beneficial.

Our understanding of mindfulness as a healing practice is grounded in over a decade of experience with thousands of people being treated for cancer and their friends and family members, as well as our personal experience with mindfulness practice. Cancer can be a profoundly lonely experience, and although each person's experience with cancer is unique, we humbly offer you the wisdom of an ancient tradition that has proven beneficial for many people like you, who have suffered with their own cancer diagnoses or those of family members or friends.

OUTLINE OF THIS BOOK

We hope to share with you our understanding of what mindfulness has to offer as a way to face cancer and support the healing process. Mindfulness is also a way of being that's endlessly enriching in and of itself. Mindfulness practice encourages you to encounter your world and your life as they unfold in the present moment, just as they are. You can apply greater awareness plus a sense of wonder, joy, and gratitude to each moment of your life. These practices reveal opportunities for growth and psychological healing that are the flip side of the traumatic cancer experiences you may have had.

In this book we will share with you the methods we teach in our Mindfulness-Based Cancer Recovery (MBCR) program in enough detail for you to develop your own practice. MBCR is the name we have given to a multifaceted eight-week program that bears a strong kinship to Jon Kabat-Zinn's Mindfulness-Based Stress Reduction (MBSR) program at the University of Massachusetts Medical Center. That MBSR program has been in operation since 1979 and served thousands of diverse patients. Initially our program for people undergoing cancer treatment was developed independently, drawing on our own experience with meditation and yoga to meet a need we saw at our local cancer center. We soon became aware of Jon Kabat-Zinn's program and adapted our format to more closely resemble his.

We did this in part to standardize our approach and to make the programs more comparable for research purposes. We also wished for people in our program to benefit from the experience that had already gone into developing and testing MBSR in Massachusetts. We have moved forward in our MBCR program with a strong research focus to better understand the effects of mindfulness and to ensure the approach's suitability for the people being treated for cancer at our center. In the chapters that follow, we will take you through our program step by step, share stories of some of the many people who have taken part in our groups, and provide specific instructions for a range of different meditation practices.

We will also address these basic questions: What is known about the complex relationship between stress and illness? What role, if any, does stress play in cancer's origins? Can stress reduction help improve outcomes for people in cancer treatment? Can it improve quality of life?

We will begin by looking at the ancient roots of mindfulness as well as the suitability of mindfulness practice to modern life. We will explore the value of mindfulness in coping with specific cancer-related issues, such as sleeping problems, pain, fatigue, stress symptoms, anxiety, and worry about the future. We will also describe a wide range of benefits that may result from mindfulness practice, from reduction of specific symptoms to possibilities for transforming yourself, your relationships, and the kind of world we are creating together. Our wish for you is that you will not only learn about mindfulness through this book, but also be empowered to apply it directly in your life each day. We hope you will not only survive your cancer experience but also, through the gifts of mindfulness, discover ways to thrive through and beyond it.

THE CANCER EXPERIENCE

Tea Ceremony
They serve tea at the cancer centre
in fine china cups
with scalloped edges
and delicate pink flowers
like the cups your grandmother used
long ago
when you were just
starting out
on your life

This long dark hallway of cancer
feels like the end
of everything

You wait
keep your eyes down
tuck into the ache of your self,

wrap your body
in the cold comfort
of fear

You will hear the tea trolley before
you see it
the fine gentle music
of tea cups and silver spoons
rattling on saucers

Take the offered cup
taste the tea
as if for the first time

This is your new life

Drink it in

—Shaun Hunter

Written by a woman in our mindfulness program, this poem describes poignantly both the fear and shock of a cancer diagnosis and also the possibilities for discovery inherent within the cancer experience. Over the course of their lives, everyone will likely be closely touched by cancer, whether through their own diagnosis or that of a family member or other loved one. From the beginning, we all dread hearing the words, "You have cancer." If you have received this diagnosis, whatever your reaction was to first hearing these words, you likely didn't hear much after that. Your mind may have raced with fears and sorrow, images of your children left behind, or painful, disfiguring treatments. You probably went on to endure a barrage of tests and treatments, waiting rooms, needles, confusing medical speak, and continued fears.

Whether you were the person diagnosed with cancer, or it was a family member or friend, your experience has likely deeply affected you.

With a cancer diagnosis comes numerous challenges. From the outset, understanding the implications and likely outcomes is difficult even for highly trained oncologists (specialist physicians who care for people with cancer). They may not have been able to exactly tell you your odds of survival. You may have found that your thoughts and feelings ran rampant with questions like "What if I don't make it?" We all see diverse media portrayals of people with cancer, ranging from the triumphant cancer patient overcoming all through sheer force of will (for example, Lance Armstrong) to the hapless and hopeless victim of pain, loss, and suffering. Unsure which group you would fall into, you may have felt as if you were on a roller-coaster ride, a wild and unsettling journey with extreme highs and lows.

Once the cancer diagnosis was confirmed, you probably had to make difficult treatment choices based on the information available, information that may have been limited or hard to understand. Studies give statistical information about prognosis or treatment effectiveness for large groups of people, but there's no way to know in advance how things will turn out for you, and this uncertainty can be maddening. Diagnostic tests and treatments can be arduous and carry their own risks. Your usual work, school, and family-life routines may have been turned upside down for a period of time, and you may have had to deal with financial hardship as a result. Your life plans and expectations may have been radically revised or put on hold as your day-to-day focus shifted to finding a way through cancer's fear and confusion. You may have found it hard at times to see a path toward recovery and return to normal life.

Treatments like surgery, chemotherapy, and radiation therapy can result in many side effects and symptoms. If you underwent an operation because of cancer, you may have had pain and discomfort and been unable to move around easily after surgery. Extreme fatigue and nausea, as well as hair loss and its resulting blow to self-esteem and identity, often accompany chemotherapy. Some people may lose all sense of taste and smell, as well as appetite. Radiation therapy can cause tenderness and burned skin near the treatment area, and the hassle of going in for daily treatments contributes to fatigue and financial burden.

After treatments are finished, people may expect you to be happy and jump right into your regular life, but this is often when you feel abandoned by the system and your care team, putting you at a crossroads in your life: what now? You may have lingering fatigue, which can last upward of a year after harsh treatments and make it nearly impossible to do much with your days. If you expected yourself to be full of energy and just happy to be alive, you may feel frustrated and disappointed if this isn't the case. Your friends and family, for their part, may seem as if they've had enough of hearing about your cancer and just want "the old you" back. If you are supporting someone who has cancer, you may also be frustrated that recovery from treatment seems to be taking so long. All of those involved are likely worried about the possibility that the cancer will come back; then what?

Yet, the possibility of losing your own or a loved one's life may serve to highlight the precious nature, vulnerability, and beauty of life itself. For many of us, a cancer diagnosis shifts what was once a vague and distant awareness of death into a very real and frightening possibility. This increased sense of mortality can be paralyzing, but it can also be a valuable catalyst for change. A cancer diagnosis can be a springboard for self-examination, personal discovery, and growth. It can provide a crucial opportunity to live life differently, intentionally, and perhaps more richly and authentically than before. The sobering wake-up call that a life crisis can represent is perhaps never more profoundly heard than following a cancer diagnosis. We have seen many people who have used the turning point that cancer provides (time off work, willingness to try new things, appreciation for the preciousness of each moment) as a chance to learn how to be more present in each moment of their lives. The results of this simple practice of mindful presence—shedding the regret, sadness, and remorse of the past and the worry, fear, and anxiety of an unknown future—can be profound. Serenity and joyful clarity of mind are sign-posts you will encounter on this path.

We invite you to sit back, take a deep breath, and begin to explore this world of mindfulness that can not only help you cope better with the challenges of living with cancer but also reveal dimensions of spaciousness and freedom from suffering you may not have known existed.

WHAT IS MINDFULNESS?

Think about what your mind is usually doing. Sometimes, it may be dwelling in the past, rehashing old events, wondering about choices you have made or how your life could have been different. You may be asking yourself, "Why did I have to get cancer? Why me? If only (this or that), maybe things would have turned out differently," which renders you sad, angry, frustrated, or remorseful. Unfortunately, you can't change the past or the fact that you are now in this situation of having to deal with cancer. This mode of thinking can only lead to more grief, but it's so hard to control. Or maybe your mind tends to race ahead with thoughts, worries, and plans about all the things that could go wrong: *What if my cancer comes back? Do I have enough money to pay the bills? How will I deal with that difficult doctor if I have to see her again?* This kind of thinking leads to even more worry, anxiety, fear, and tension in the body. But for the moment, these future scenarios are imaginary, made up by your active mind. Mark Twain is credited with the quote, "My life has been a series of tragedies; most of them never happened."

So while you are ruminating about the past, worrying about potential hazards in the future, or simply losing yourself in a maze of conflicting thoughts and concerns, you miss the only time you can actually live in: the present. If you think about it, you'll see that everything happens only in the present moment. Ruminating about the past or worrying about the future happens now, but while you are doing that, you miss all the other things that are also occurring now: a conversation with a friend, a flower's blooming, a blue sky, and a cool breeze. You also miss cues your body may be sending you: tension in your shoulders and neck, tightness in your belly, a sense of fullness or hunger—information that helps you respond to your body's needs. If you can't live fully now, in the present moment, when can you? There's no time to live other than now, and no matter what difficult events happened in the past or may happen in the future, often in the present moment, things are just fine or at least quite bearable. As John Newton stated, "We can easily manage if we will only take, each day, the burden appointed to it. But the load will be too heavy for us if we carry yesterday's burden over again today, and then add the burden of the morrow before we are required to bear it."

People with cancer have told us about bumping into friends after diagnosis who say something like "You look so good." It happens often enough that one person with cancer had buttons created with that slogan as a kind of inside joke she shared with her support group. After all, how should she look? When you think about it, the major change that occurs between the day before diagnosis and the day after has to do with the meaning of the diagnosis for the future, and this is where the mind holds sway. It seems to be the case that if you can be present for your life as it actually occurs, much of the angst of the past and future simply falls away. It may seem hard to believe, but this is possible even in the midst of a life crisis like cancer.

We once heard a story of a meditation retreat held by Jon Kabat-Zinn, the founder of the MBSR program: there was a large clock on the wall of the meditation hall; he covered it up with a big sign that simply read "NOW." The time is *always* now; that's all you need to know. So mindfulness is a way of being in which you are awake and aware of the present moment. It also incorporates the way in which you pay attention, which is the attitudinal component of mindfulness. You pay attention in a nonjudgmental, accepting, open, and curious way. This attitude allows you smile and shake your head when you notice your mind wandering, as if you were watching a rather cute puppy's antics, rather than beating yourself with a mental stick. So mindfulness is simple: pay attention to whatever comes up in the present moment; allow it all to rise and fall of its own accord, without trying to change anything; and be with things as they are. Though simple, the concept is by no means easy in practice. Many people spend a lifetime trying to refine these skills. It's said that a journey of a thousand miles begins with a single step; in terms of beginning this particular journey, we would only add: there's no time like the present!

ROOTS OF MINDFULNESS

We have already said a fair bit about mindfulness, but little about meditation and how the two relate to each other. Though there are many different forms of meditation, a shared feature of most is that awareness is directed toward a particular object or aspect of experience. In a basic sense, meditation means purposefully paying close attention to something and sustaining that attention for a period of time. The reasons suggested for paying attention in this way include developing concentration or stability of mind; creating conditions favorable to tranquility or peace; and developing greater insight, understanding, and compassion.

Approaches to meditation emphasizing mindfulness instruct us to direct the mind's attending, observing, and knowing powers toward not only external events and bodily experience as revealed through the senses, but also the activities of the mind itself. Through this practice, we can become more familiar with how the mind works, its role in creating and shaping our experience, and its potential contribution to health and healing. This direct knowing of the way things work is an invaluable asset for successfully navigating the challenges of illness.

Long before the development of modern scientific methods, people set out to understand the nature of reality using basic tools such as observation, analysis, and contemplation. In India, on the Himalayan plateau, and in ancient China, a number of philosophical traditions developed, systematically exploring important questions that still have relevance for us today. Among them are questions about the causes of health and illness and the nature of human suffering.

Yoga and Buddhism, two traditions that are close cousins, developed theories of the mind and meditative practices that speak as clearly to our modern-day troubles as they did to those of southern Asia twenty-five hundred years ago. For those unfamiliar with the story of Siddhartha Gautama's enlightenment and how he became the historical Buddha or "awakened one," it may be helpful to share it briefly here.

According to tradition, Siddhartha was born to an influential family and had a princely upbringing. At his birth it was prophesied that he would become either a great king or a holy man. His father, who preferred that his son follow a royal destiny, took pains to shield Siddhartha from knowledge of human suffering, illness, old age, death, and religious teachings that might awaken him to spiritual or philosophical concerns. Despite those efforts, at the age of twenty-nine, Siddhartha chanced upon an old man and learned that everyone eventually becomes old and frail. This upset the young prince but also spurred him to explore the world further; as a result he encountered sickness and death. He decided to leave the confines of his home and, for six years, pursued the life of a wandering holy man, begging alms and engaging in extreme austerities, such as fasting and walking long distances, which eventually left him near death.

At that point he chose to reconsider his path, because he didn't see the value of such extreme self-sacrifice. He recalled a time from his childhood when he had sat under a tree, watching his father lead a ceremony that marked the beginning of the growing season. While peacefully enjoying the day, he had spontaneously entered a calm and blissful state. He now came to wonder if that long-ago experience could contain a key to the understanding he was seeking. Following this lead, he adopted "the middle way," a path that avoids the extreme of either self-indulgence or self-denial. Further, through entering and deepening his meditation, he came to a full understanding of the causes of human suffering and the way to end it, which forms the core of his teaching.

We share this story because we think it's important to acknowledge our debt to the original sources of the methods we will share with you. We want to make it clear, though, that you don't have to be a Buddhist or to even have read or studied Buddhism to follow the program we are setting out. It's compatible with many worldviews. Indeed, most spiritual and religious traditions have some element of meditation or mindfulness embedded in their traditional practices. The approach we present is entirely secular; by "secular" we don't mean rejecting of religion or spirituality but, rather, accepting of all faith traditions. We have had program participants from diverse backgrounds who have been able to fit these methods into their own belief systems.

Although this program is based on practices with ancient roots, we encourage you not to unquestioningly accept what we share. We are committed to subjecting these methods and the whole approach to the rigors of science, and we hope that on a personal level, you, too, will put the practices to the test in your own life. It might even help to adopt a stance of open-minded skepticism. We expect that you will discover through experience, as we have, that "the proof is in the pudding."

DEVELOPMENT OF MBCR

It might help to relate to you in a bit more detail how our program came to be. In 1995, having worked as a newly minted psychologist for a couple of years, I (Michael) found myself working in a busy cancer treatment center in Calgary, Alberta. One day, two colleagues and I were sitting together having lunch in the hospital cafeteria and talking about our work, which consisted primarily of counseling and providing support to people in cancer treatment and their families.

While discussing, with some awe and not a little reverence, the immense challenges many people undergoing cancer treatment encounter and often overcome, we also spoke of our gratitude for the opportunity to do the work we did. Eventually we got around to acknowledging that this work was not without cost to us. Caring about the people with whom we worked meant sharing in their losses and grief as well as their triumphs. These experiences also heightened our own sense of vulnerability. As our discussion deepened, we discovered that we had something else in common. Each of us, to some degree, relied on meditation and yoga to cope with the stresses of our own lives. It occurred to us that some of our patients might benefit from these practices in a different way than counseling could provide. We wondered if it would be possible for us to offer a program where we could share what we had learned through our own experience with meditation. How would it be accepted in the highly technical and institutional medical setting that was our workplace?

From that point on, we set out to develop a program. We cobbled together bits and pieces of the yoga and meditation we had practiced, and we tied it into what we knew about stress and the mind-body perspective from our training as health professionals. From this, we created a workbook for participants. There were about equal parts yoga, including yogic breathing practices, and a range of meditation techniques, including mindfulness meditation. The first few times we ran the program, we obtained written feedback from everyone at the end of what were then seven-week sessions, and we used that information to refine our approach. Word quickly spread, and we had little difficulty filling our classes.

Along the way we became aware of Jon Kabat-Zinn and his MBSR approach. We developed a profound respect for the sensitivity and thoroughness with which he had described his work in his book *Full Catastrophe Living: Using the Wisdom of Your Mind and Body to Face Stress, Pain, and Illness* (Kabat-Zinn 1990), and began to recommend it to all of our patients. At about that time, in 1996 to 1997, we began to implement a formal study comparing the changes over time between patients randomized to either our mindfulness program or a wait-list control condition, and Linda joined our team as a clinician and researcher. We were pleased to find that the outcomes of that study supported our impressions of the value of these methods and the participants' reports of benefit.

The results were published in the journal *Psychosomatic Medicine* in 2000 (Speca et al. 2000) and, since then, have been cited hundreds of times in the scientific literature. The first to systematically evaluate mindfulness meditation for people with cancer, we ourselves were surprised by the amount of improvement seen in the people who took the program compared to those who were still waiting. Overall, people who took the program had a 65 percent reduction in total mood disturbance, which included measures of anxiety, depression, and anger (Speca et al. 2000). They also felt more vigorous, and less fatigued and confused. They had an overall 35 percent reduction in stress symptoms, including decreased muscle tension, stomach and bowel problems, and nervous system arousal, as well as reduced irritability and habitual stress reactions, such as sleep problems, overeating, and drinking (ibid.). These benefits persisted up to six months later (Carlson et al. 2001). We went on to conduct many more studies, which you can access online, but this was the beginning of the story of MBCR, which continues today.

IS MINDFULNESS FOR YOU?

Our objective throughout this book is to point out ways we have learned that will help you become more mindful of your experience as it happens and respond to life stressors in skillful and positive ways. After laying out the MBCR program, we will introduce you to the core concepts of mindfulness and practices that will gradually allow you to increase your ability to pay attention to the present moment. You could certainly just read the book and leave it at that, which you would likely enjoy. At the same time, the heart of the practice is just that: practice. If you don't commit to regular practice, you aren't likely to see much substantial change in your life. So we challenge you to make this commitment: can you set aside some time for yourself every day, just for your own healing and well-being? Can you make this a priority, at least for a reasonable trial period? If you are willing to approach this practice with an open mind and heart, and try what we suggest, amazing things can happen. If you are skeptical, that's okay. Please try the program and see for yourself. In the words of the Buddha:

> Do not believe in anything simply because you have heard it.
>
> Do not believe in anything simply because it is spoken and rumored by many.
>
> Do not believe in anything simply because it is found written in your religious books.

Do not believe in anything merely on the authority of your teachers and elders.

Do not believe in traditions because they have been handed down for many generations.

But after observation and analysis, when you find that anything agrees with reason

and is conducive to the good and benefit of one and all,

accept it and live up to it.

CHAPTER 2

Stress and Cancer

Grant that I may be given appropriate difficulties and sufferings on this journey so that my heart can be truly awakened and my practice of liberation and universal compassion may be truly fulfilled.

—Traditional Tibetan prayer

Some of the first things that come to mind for many people with cancer when they hear that we run a stress reduction program are that maybe stress caused their cancer, maybe it was all their fault, and therefore maybe it's now their job to beat the cancer by changing the way they face stress. This way of viewing cancer is not accurate and, in our opinion, not very helpful either. Isn't it bad enough that you are facing this illness in the first place? The last thing you need on top of that is to feel guilty about it. However, there are things you can do to help right now. In this chapter we will share with you a bit of background about stress: what it is, its purpose, and how you can detect it, as well as a more thorough overview of whether, and to what extent, stress or other psychological factors play a role in cancer's development or progression. We intend to present the scientific evidence in a way that, while not overly simplistic, doesn't get into minutiae. We'd like you to take what's helpful from this discussion and use it as a springboard to do what you can to improve the quality of your life in the here and now, no matter what you are dealing with.

THE STRESS RESPONSE

Understanding what happens in your body when you are in a situation you perceive as stressful is very important, so you can start becoming aware of when this is happening and learn to turn down the stress response when it isn't necessary or helpful to you. You may have heard of "fight or flight." This refers to that instantaneous surge of energy you feel when confronted by a real danger, like almost getting into a car accident. Your heart races, your breath quickens, and you may break out in a thin layer of cold sweat and feel your stomach churning. Your body is preparing to either fight off the danger or flee for safety. This system of arousal enables us to deal effectively with acute threats to survival. It relies on a complex cascade of events involving the nerves and hormones. When you perceive a threat, your brain immediately sends signals to your nervous system and hormonal system that result in the release of various chemicals throughout the body; you have likely heard of adrenaline, also called epinephrine, which is one of these.

These chemicals trigger the various symptoms that accompany the stress reaction, including increased blood pressure, quickened pulse and heart rate, a rush of blood away from the torso to the limbs (to allow for fast running), sharpened mental focus and vision (to better see the danger), and a "hold" on mundane housekeeping tasks like digesting food (this can wait for safety). The stress response affects the whole body, by way of complex and interconnected processes involving multiple systems, including the nervous, hormonal, and immune systems. The whole thing is triggered almost instantaneously, as you will recall if you've ever had to jump out the way of a speeding car. It also usually resolves back to a normal, calm state shortly after the threat has passed.

Now this would be all well and good if the stressors encountered in daily life were all saber-toothed tigers or even speeding cars, but it's not so simple in modern times. The threats tigers or speeding cars pose are very discrete: they happen, are dealt with one way or another, then are put behind us. Normally, when the threat is gone, the system allows the "relaxation response" to replace this whole cascade of the stress response so that the opposite of stress activation occurs: your pulse slows down, your breathing goes back to normal, your digestion and elimination proceed, you can get back to eating and sleeping, and healing is facilitated.

Unfortunately, the stressors in modern life are rarely so straightforward: they are things like constant job pressure and tight deadlines, arguments with your kids or spouse, financial worries, heavy traffic and rude drivers, fear of crime and terrorism, and, for the cancer survivor, fear of sometimes painful and debilitating treatments and disease recurrence. But even though the stressors today are different and typically not life threatening, our bodies react similarly to the way they would when encountering the short-term life-threatening dangers the system is designed to help us with.

Perhaps even reading the previous list of troubles has resulted in a stress reaction in your body. You get wired up to either fight or flee, but in modern society, there's rarely a dramatic action that will resolve these problems or discharge the energy of this reaction. Sure, you can hit your boss, but probably only once! Then what? Running away from your spouse might do for one or two arguments, but it's not going to solve the larger problem. So what can you do? Your body reacts to stressful situations with a flood of hormones that might help you to cope in certain situations, but modern stressors are everywhere (at least it can seem that way). So it's possible to be in a state of high arousal, a low-level fight-or-flight reaction, almost all the time, which can carry on to the point of exhaustion. Imagine the wear and tear this can cause.

THE EFFECTS OF PROLONGED STRESS

Indeed, ample research shows physical effects of high stress levels and prolonged exposure to stressors on a wide variety of symptoms and medical conditions. For example, in Pittsburgh, research psychologist Sheldon Cohen (2005) investigated the effects of stress on the common cold and flu. To control for a wide variety of variables that might affect who gets sick and when, he went so far as to take a group of volunteers and inject them with identical flu viruses. He then had them stay in quarantine in dormitory-style housing for a week, eating the same foods and doing the same things, and looked at who got the flu and how bad it was. He even had them save in zipper-locked plastic bags all the tissues they used to blow their noses, and he weighed the tissues to see how much mucus was excreted. He also asked the subjects to assess their stress levels in a variety of ways before they were exposed to the viruses. What he found verified the results of other studies done in people's own homes: those who had higher stress levels before exposure to the virus were more likely to have flu and cold symptoms, and they secreted more mucus. When Cohen analyzed what types of stressors were most likely to cause colds and flu, two stood out: interpersonal problems with family and friends, and work problems (being unemployed or working a job that was below the person's level of training or experience). Both of these are often chronic and ongoing life stressors.

So the story from this and other careful research is that short-term stress isn't necessarily harmful, so long as it can be dealt with and you soon return to a baseline state of relative calm. However, if you are exposed to prolonged life stress and can't bring your body back into harmony, you may be more susceptible to a wide variety of physical and emotional illnesses. Later in this chapter we will discuss what this means specifically for cancer, because the story isn't as simple as for the common cold.

RECOGNIZING YOUR STRESS SYMPTOMS

The physiological stress response results in a range of symptoms, but psychological stress can also manifest in a wide variety of ways. Take a moment to complete the following checklist, "Symptoms of Stress Self-Assessment."

SYMPTOMS OF STRESS SELF-ASSESSMENT

Check off any of the following stress symptoms you experienced in the last week:

Physical Symptoms

☐ Headaches   ☐ Sleep difficulties   ☐ Racing heart

☐ Indigestion   ☐ Dizziness   ☐ Restlessness

☐ Stomachaches   ☐ Back pain   ☐ Tiredness

☐ Sweaty palms   ☐ Tight neck and   ☐ Ringing in ears
                       shoulders

Behavioral Symptoms

☐ Smoking   ☐ Grinding teeth at night

☐ Bossiness   ☐ Overuse of alcohol

☐ Compulsive gum chewing   ☐ Compulsive eating

☐ Critical attitude   ☐ Inability to get things done

Emotional Symptoms

☐ Crying   ☐ Overwhelming feeling of

☐ Nervousness, anxiety   pressure

☐ Boredom, no meaning to   ☐ Anger
   things   ☐ Loneliness

☐ Edginess, ready to explode   ☐ Unhappiness for no reason

☐ Feeling powerless to change   ☐ Easily upset
   things

Cognitive Symptoms

☐ Trouble thinking clearly   ☐ Indecisiveness

☐ Forgetfulness   ☐ Thoughts of running away

☐ Lack of creativity   ☐ Constant worry

☐ Memory loss   ☐ Loss of sense of humor

Spiritual Symptoms

☐ Emptiness   ☐ Martyrdom   ☐ Cynicism
☐ Loss of meaning ☐ Apathy   ☐ Unforgiving of
☐ Doubt   ☐ Loss of direction   self and others
                                     ☐ Need to prove
                                        self

Relational Symptoms

☐ Isolation   ☐ Hiding   ☐ Lack of intimacy
☐ Intolerance   ☐ Clamming up   ☐ Using people
☐ Resentment   ☐ Lowered sex   ☐ Fewer contacts
☐ Loneliness   drive   with friends
☐ Distrust   ☐ Nagging   ☐ Lashing out

What did you notice as you completed the checklist? For one thing, you probably saw that the symptoms are divided into a number of different categories. You probably also noticed that though you could check off a few items in each area, one or more areas predominated. Maybe you surprised yourself at the high number of check marks on the page! What's important to take from this exercise is getting acquainted with *your* personal patterns of stress reacting. Everyone is different. For example, Margaret is a breast-cancer survivor who found herself checking off many of the physical and emotional symptoms of stress: she gets headaches, has trouble sleeping, has tight neck and shoulder muscles, and sometimes feels a bit dizzy. She also feels nervous, worries a lot, and finds it hard to concentrate or make decisions, even about the smallest things. She is forgetful and often feels overwhelmed by life's everyday demands.

In contrast, Michael, a lymphoma survivor, has stress symptoms that are more likely to affect his behavior and relationships. He finds himself clamming up, keeping to himself and withdrawing from friends and family, drinking alcohol to help get to sleep at night, and grinding his teeth. Often irritable, he lashes out at his wife and kids for no real reason.

Both of these people may be experiencing similar stressors in their lives, but they have learned to react differently. Identifying your characteristic pattern of stress reacting helps you become more aware of instances when you need to take action.

WHERE DOES STRESS COME FROM?

It's neither fun nor healthy to experience stress symptoms for long periods of time. The good news is that you have a degree of choice in the matter. Where does stress comes from? You might say it's out there in the world—in the doctor's appointments, demanding bosses, credit card companies, and speeding cars—but that's not actually true. The stress comes from *inside you*, from that part of you that decides whether or not something's a problem. That's not to say that receiving a cancer diagnosis and having to deal with all that goes with it isn't a huge difficulty; we would never deny that it is. *But* have you ever noticed that some people deal with life challenges in a calmer and more assured way than others? How do they do that? Part of the answer is that they *interpret* the meaning of these life events differently; they have likely learned a range of specific skills to help them cope, and perhaps most important, they have a sense of trust or confidence that they can deal pretty effectively with whatever arises.

We will discuss some of this further in this chapter and in much more detail throughout the book, but here are two key points:

1. The first step in changing your stress reactions is to become aware of them, to learn to recognize them in action: the how, when, and why they show up in your life.

2. The next step is understanding that you have a choice in how you respond to and deal with life events.

Mindfulness practice will help tremendously in both regards.

STRESS AND THE MIND-BODY CONNECTION

At this point it helps to clarify what we mean when we speak of "the mind" and "mindfulness" and how they relate to stress. A common assumption is that the mind is what we think with or, from the medical-science viewpoint, the working of our brains. You may have heard something about the "mind-body problem"; in brief, this has to do with the nature of consciousness and its relationship to our physical bodies. It's not our purpose to fully answer these questions, which puzzle scientists and philosophers to this day. Rather, for the sake of clarity, we would like to develop a shared practical understanding with you of these terms as we use them.

When we refer to the mind, we are not solely or even primarily concerned with thinking or cognition. As a T-shirt slogan proclaims, "Meditation…it's not what you think!" Rather, we are concerned with a range of processes and subjective experiences, including perception, thought, and emotion, and even our basic capacity to know anything at all. We could say that mind is consciousness as embodied and experienced, in our case, by human beings. What we think of as mind and body are in fact a functional unity; that is, they work together, never separately. Neither mind and body nor thoughts and feelings exist or function independently of each other in real living, breathing organisms. So it just doesn't make sense to separate them practically; when we think, we feel, and each process influences the other.

While this way of thinking about the mind is foreign to some traditional approaches to science, it likely fits nicely with your own experience. Take a moment to remember some pleasant experience from a joyful time in your life, maybe when you participated in an activity or spent time with friends and family. As you do so, you may see the events replayed in your mind's eye; you can probably describe the experience in words and concepts; and if the memory is vivid enough, you likely experience in your body a felt sense of the associated emotions, such as joy and happiness. At another level, if we used the proper tools, we would discover that this reexperiencing of events mentally correlates with subtle neurological and physiological changes throughout your body.

24

One implication of these changes is that we can experience stress and very strong emotional reactions based primarily on our own thoughts rather than ongoing external events. For example, imagine sucking on a tart lemon wedge. As you imagine this, you may notice your mouth puckering and even some salivation; but there are likely no lemons present as you read this, so how does this reaction happen? Similar cause-and-effect relationships exist between more-complex mental events and physical changes in our bodies. Critical judgments about ourselves or worry about feared future events can have very real consequences for our well-being in the here and now, because our bodies respond to these mind events almost as if they were really happening.

Bodymind and *heartmind* are two terms that have been used to try to capture this unity. Whether or not you choose to use these terms, recognizing the interplay and mutual influence between mental and emotional events and the physical body is critical for understanding the stress response. It will also allow you to recognize how your thinking and behavior can create more-favorable conditions to health and happiness.

MINDFULNESS AND STRESS

So how does mindfulness fit in with all this? We began to describe mindfulness in chapter 1. Now let's consider why it matters in a practical sense in relation to the day-to-day stresses we encounter. Recall that mindfulness refers to being intentionally aware—that is, paying attention. In particular, it means intentionally noticing what you are experiencing and your reactions to your experience—perceptions, thoughts, and feelings—as they occur in the present moment, moment by moment. To the degree that you are mindful of your reactions to stresses as they occur, you gain opportunities to modify your response. For example, suppose a rude driver cuts you off in traffic and then gestures and shouts out the window at you. Your first instinctive reaction may be to defend yourself and shout right back; after all, you did nothing wrong. However, you could also think, *Wow, this person is really miserable and taking it out on a complete stranger; do I want to be like that too?* You might then feel some sympathy; take the high road; and with a smile and wave, allow the rude driver to pull in front of you.

If you become aware of habitual patterns that amplify your stress, you can choose to sidestep these knee-jerk reactions. The first step in any process of change is awareness, which mindfulness practice allows us to cultivate. Bringing greater awareness to a situation, *in and of itself,* may help us refrain from making things worse through our reactions. It also allows us to access a broader range of inner resources in that moment, to respond more creatively and in ways that honor our deeper wisdom and aspirations. We will discuss this in more detail in chapter 4. The main thing to understand now is that you have an innate capacity for mindfulness that can be developed and strengthened through specific meditation practices we will share with you in this book.

STRESS AND CANCER

Earlier in this chapter we outlined some research showing that prolonged stress can lead to a higher likelihood of getting colds and the flu. People have also been interested in the question of whether stress plays some role in cancer's onset and progression. To get to the point, the answer right now is that we don't really know, but there are some interesting nuances you might like to hear about. Typically this type of research looks at whether stress is related to cancer incidence (who gets cancer) or progression (once you have cancer, what is its course).

Stress and Cancer Incidence

Imagine how you might try to answer the question: does stress cause cancer? You could ask a bunch of people who got cancer, "Were you stressed before you got sick?" and then compare their answers to those of people who didn't get cancer, but you can see how this might be problematic. Surely if someone asked us that question, we would say, "Well, yes, I sure must have been stressed; after all, I got cancer!" In fact we know from careful research that this kind of biased recall is exactly what happens. Also consider, what if the events in question happened years earlier? How could you even remember what was really going on? So that retrospective technique doesn't work.

A better approach would be to gather a big group of people, assuming that in time some of them would go on to contract various illnesses, and ask them a lot of questions. You would want to ask about their stress levels, their mood, family history of illness, and other risk factors for cancer, and then just wait to see what happened. Of course, you would have to wait for a very long time to get a large enough group who were diagnosed with cancer, and it would be expensive to do. Then you would have to be very careful to take into account all the other known risk factors for cancer, especially since some of them are also associated with higher stress levels or certain personality traits, including things like diet, smoking, drinking alcohol, physical activity, exposure to environmental and occupational carcinogens, family history, and genetics. Perhaps you can begin to see that this type of study is difficult, time consuming, and expensive!

Nonetheless, several big studies of this nature have been conducted and reviewed. In his paper, "Psychological Factors and Cancer Development: Evidence After 30 Years of Research," Bert Garssen (2004) summarized only those superior studies that used prospective designs with proper controls, as described previously. Seventy studies were included in the review. Garssen broke down the vague category of "stress" into discrete dimensions that were often measured in these studies. The areas of interest were stressful life events (including a wide range of events like divorce, illness, and job loss right down to holidays and children leaving home); loss events (losing a child or spouse); social support; quality of partner relationship; personality; coping styles; and measures of distress, depression, and psychiatric diagnoses. Each of these factors had been theorized to potentially impact cancer development.

So what did Garssen find? There was no clear evidence that stressful life events, bereavement and loss, social relations or distress, and depression symptoms were related to getting cancer, even though in each area several studies did find a relationship between a given factor and cancer. For example, of fourteen studies that looked at whether depression levels predicted later cancer onset, seven found that depression *did* predict cancer initiation, but seven found that depression *did not*! This shows how important it is to review a whole body of literature, rather than just rely on one or two studies. Whichever view you hold, there's research available to support your contention.

Stress and Cancer Survival

The picture is a bit clearer, however, when we turn to the question of whether stress or other psychological factors play a role in survival once cancer has been diagnosed. Perhaps you can imagine that this type of study would be easier to conduct. The number of people you need to study is smaller than in a study of cancer incidence, and the time necessary for the study is usually shorter. You still have to control for myriad background factors that may be important and, in addition, consider the types of treatments received and the nature of the cancer itself (the size of the tumor, stage, grade, node status, spread, and so on), as well as the type of cancer, since cancers do not all behave in the same way.

For example, breast cancer is an endocrine-sensitive cancer that's influenced by hormones. If stress affects hormone levels, we may hypothesize that it affects the outcome of hormonally mediated cancers, such as breast or prostate cancer, but not types that aren't as hormonally responsive, such as lung or brain cancer. Similarly, diet affects colorectal cancer, and smoking affects lung cancer, so these factors must be taken into account, especially if people with higher stress levels or depression are also more likely to smoke or have poor eating habits. You can see how it might be possible to conclude that people with lung cancer with more depression died sooner than those with less depression, when in reality the reason they died sooner is that they were heavier smokers (who also happened to be more depressed)! Good studies attempt to take all of this into consideration, but you can imagine how hard that is to do when there are many factors affecting survival.

That said, some evidence suggests that a few psychological factors may be important for survival after cancer diagnosis, including social support. In a 1995 study by Elizabeth Maunsell and colleagues in Montreal, 224 women with recently diagnosed breast cancer were asked whether they had a confidant with whom they had discussed personal problems in the three months since surgery. Researchers then followed the women for seven years, controlled for a wide variety of medical and psychological factors, and found the survival rate in women without a confidant to be 56 percent, compared to 72 percent for women who'd had at least one type of confidant (such as a spouse, child, friend, colleague, or health professional) (Maunsell, Brisson, and Deschênes 1995). This finding suggests that it's a good idea to share your burden with other important people in your life.

You may also have read in other books or magazines about research into the importance of certain coping styles, such as the "fighting spirit." In a 1979 study, Stephen Greer and colleagues found that women who had a coping style of fighting spirit or denial survived longer than those who reacted with either stoic acceptance or a helpless attitude (Greer, Morris, and Pettingale 1979). However, these findings have not been replicated in many other studies over the years. One of Greer's findings may still hold, though: six of ten studies in the Garssen review (2004) found that helplessness and hopelessness, or pessimism, were associated with unfavorable disease course.

So what do we make of all this? Should everyone just "put on a happy face" and get on with it? That's certainly not our stance. We know that false expression of emotions is not helpful, either psychologically or physically. It's normal to feel distressed, depressed, and even hopeless at times when dealing with cancer. We do not advocate that you just "stay positive" and force aside the unhappy thoughts.

Another research finding that's important here is that emotional repression and suppression have also been associated with poorer cancer prognosis. In the Garssen review (2004), the role of repression in cancer progression is demonstrated in five out of eight studies. *Emotional repression* is the denial of negative emotions, even to yourself, while *suppression* is the purposeful shoving down of negative and difficult emotions you don't want to have, deal with, or let others see you experiencing. All of these behaviors seem to have a negative influence on survival outcomes. Of course, the data isn't conclusive, but it supports what we, as longtime psychologists, well know. People do better and feel better when they can openly express whatever emotions are troubling them, work though them, resolve problems, and perhaps reach a place of peace and equanimity. We have seen many people realize this possibility, even in the face of cancer.

But what if you do all you can and your cancer continues to progress? Is it your fault for not trying hard enough? Absolutely not. There are many factors involved in cancer progression that even cancer biologists and oncologists don't understand, and over which you have little or no control. At a minimum, the type of cancer, its size, its aggressiveness, your family history, the treatments you received, and how well you tolerated them all play a role.

One thing we do know is that the quality of life, regardless of duration, matters a great deal. The quality of your life depends to a large degree on choices for which you do have responsibility. For this, you can be grateful. Whether you will live for days, months, or many years, you have an opportunity to make the very best of it. If coping well and living mindfully help you to live longer by some as yet uncertain mechanisms, wonderful.

COPING WITH STRESS

Earlier we discussed the idea that stress reactions were unique to each person and that some people seemed to cope better with difficult life situations than others. One reason for this is that the people who cope better may be using more-effective coping styles or the right coping style at the right time. We'd like to emphasize a couple of points here. The first is that no one coping style will be effective in all situations. The second is that the match between the demands of the situation and the approach to coping is of utmost importance.

One helpful way to think about life events is to divide them into things that are largely controllable and things that are largely uncontrollable. For example, you can't control whether or not a traffic jam happens, but you can control whether you leave early for work if you think traffic will likely be heavy. The best approach to dealing with controllable versus uncontrollable events is also different. When you have some degree of control over events, the best coping style is *problem-focused coping*, which simply means doing something to solve the problem. If the problem is that you tend to be late for work, try getting up earlier, arranging your clothes and briefcase the night before, preparing as well as you can so no one delays you at home, and leaving early enough to get there on time even if you happen to encounter slow traffic.

If the problem is not controllable, the best approach is often *emotion-focused coping*, which means you deal with the emotions the stressor brought up, since you can't change the situation itself. An example of a situation that's not under your control may be having to wait hours for a doctor's appointment. As a cancer patient or support person, you've likely experienced the scenario of sitting in the waiting room for quite a while since your appointment time, waiting and getting more and more anxious and frustrated when your name is not called: *What is wrong with these people? What can I do to speed things up? I have things to do, places to go; I can't sit here all day!* You can get yourself more and more riled up, but what use is that? You'll be sitting there for just as long whether you're happy or miserable. Now is the time to note your emotions as they arise, using mindfulness skills and applying strategies to deal with these uncomfortable feelings.

So much of the cancer journey is uncontrollable and unpredictable. Most people have well-developed problem-solving skills, but fewer know how to cope with the unknown and the uncontrollable. We will devote much of this book to teaching you how to do just that.

PART II

The MBCR Program

CHAPTER 3

Beginning the Program

Now that you have some background about the origins and philosophy behind the MBCR program, it's time to begin the nuts and bolts of learning mindfulness practice. It helps to think of mindfulness in two ways, which we often call "big-M mindfulness" and "little-m mindfulness" (Shapiro and Carlson 2009). The big "M" refers to mindfulness as a way of being in the world that spans all that you do every moment of your life; you can be mindful or not. It's not specific to any activity or situation. In contrast, little-m mindfulness refers to purposefully setting aside a chunk of time in your day to practice being mindful, just as you would practice the piano if you wished to learn that skill. Mindfulness is also a skill that you learn only through repeated doing. Essentially you practice little-m mindfulness to make it possible to be more mindful in the world (the big "M"). It's virtually impossible to achieve big-M mindfulness without a very strong and regular little-m practice. So that's where we will start.

INTENTION, ATTENTION, AND ATTITUDE

If you are reading this book, you obviously have an interest in learning mindfulness meditation. You may have been drawn to it because you are suffering acutely from stress, fatigue, pain, or nausea. You may be suffering in other ways, with depression, anxiety, or worry about your future, or have a general sense that life could just be better or more meaningful. It's helpful at this point to ask yourself, *Why do I want to do this? What's my intention behind learning mindfulness meditation?* Research on meditation has shown that people generally get out if it what they intend to, and intentions often shift over time: In a group of experienced meditators, Deane Shapiro found that intentions shifted from self-regulation to self-exploration, and finally to self-liberation and service to others (Shapiro 1992). Those whose goal was regulation of emotions and stress management attained that goal, and those whose goal was self-exploration and transcendence beyond the self moved in that direction.

We looked at this issue in cancer survivors by interviewing people in our drop-in groups who had practiced meditation for several years (Mackenzie et al. 2007). At first they told us the practice was used to control specific symptoms, such as tension and stress, but later on, the focus became more about spirituality and personal growth. It may help to consider intention as a direction rather than a destination.

Along these lines, I (Linda), with Shauna Shapiro and others, published a paper proposing a model we called "IAA," for intention, attention, and attitude (Shapiro et al. 2006). The "I" is your intention, or motivation, for meditating. We emphasized the importance of thinking about your intention before you begin a course of practice. This may change over time and could range widely, from *I intend to make the world a better place for all beings* to *I intend to learn to notice when I experience stress symptoms, and let them go.* An additional benefit of clarifying your reasons for meditating is that it boosts your motivation. It's easier to make a commitment and expend effort toward something when you remind yourself of its importance to you. While it's important to consider your overall intention or motivation, you then need to step back so that you can apply the attitude of nonstriving to your practice, as described next. The first "A" in the model refers to attention, which is the most obvious element of mindfulness practice; you have to pay attention before anything else can happen. The second "A" refers to the attitudes you apply to the endeavor, which are also crucial to ensure a warm and nurturing practice, rather than one that's harsh, cold, or disciplinarian.

Helpful Attitudes

As you prepare to launch into mindfulness practice, it's very important to keep in mind not only why you want to practice (your intention) and the logistics of what to do (pay attention), but also the way you approach them. There's a range of attitudes that are helpful to adopt, including nonjudgment, which we mentioned in chapter 1, and others that are meant to create an atmosphere that's friendly, curious, and open to whatever arises.

It's also important to be flexible and accepting of your limitations and the conditions the nature of the world itself imposes. We like to use the metaphor of training a puppy: when the puppy wanders off, you kindly and gently lead it back to its path, while smiling and shaking your head at its cute and sometimes-silly antics. You know the puppy is just being a puppy, and you can't blame it for that. The same goes with minds: they wander, jump around, and generally misbehave all the time. That's just the way they are; we're willing to bet yours is no exception. They may even mess in the corner on occasion (both our minds and puppies!); it's tempting to get really mad and frustrated, but if you've had a puppy, you know that the best response is consistent, kind attention. The same truly does apply to minds (and hearts).

You are about to begin a program of training your mind, body, and heart to a new way of being. It's simple, but by no means easy. Many people spend a lifetime refining these skills. The attitudes outlined next, based on those Jon Kabat-Zinn suggested in his excellent book *Full Catastrophe Living* (Kabat-Zinn 1990), will help you as you begin this journey.

Nonjudgment: Mindfulness is cultivated by assuming a gentle stance of impartial witness to your own experience. This requires that you become aware of the constant stream of evaluative and judgmental thoughts you have, and then try to step back. With a nonjudging mind, things are neither "good" nor "bad," but simply the way they are.

Patience: Patience demonstrates that you understand and accept that things have their own schedule for unfolding. People tend to be particularly impatient with themselves, expecting that they "should" be able to calm the mind, stop the thoughts, or get over whatever's upsetting them. Nature has a "mind of its own," and patience allows you to simply observe the unfolding of the bodymind over time.

Beginner's mind: To see the richness of the present moment, it helps to cultivate a mind that's willing and able to see everything as if for the very first time. If you think you know it all, then there's nothing left to discover. With beginner's mind, the joys of the world as they unfold around us become new again, as if we were all children, freed from our old expectations.

Trust: Living in a world of experts can lead you to begin doubting yourself. Innately you are the best expert on you; for matters of personal growth, it's far better to open to your own feelings and intuition than to get caught up in outside authorities. In meditation practice, if something doesn't feel right to you, pay attention and examine your feelings. Trust in your intuition and your own basic wisdom, goodness, and ability to work through challenges.

Nonstriving: Mindfulness meditation is different from other human activity; we do it not with a goal or destination in mind, but rather with a mind toward simply being, not doing. There's no goal other than for you to be conscious of yourself as you are. The paradoxical aspect of meditation practice is that only by truly letting go of striving toward a goal or outcome will you potentially reach that outcome.

Acceptance: Acceptance involves seeing things as they actually are. You may not like it, but if that's the way things are, so they are. Acknowledging the truth of your life is the first step in any genuine process of change. Through acceptance, you cease struggling to change things that are beyond your ability to control, and you free yourself from the weight of denial.

Letting go: Letting go, also known as "nonattachment," is fundamental to mindfulness practice. It involves recognizing and welcoming the ever-changing nature of experience. The human tendency to hold on to some parts of our experience and reject others is a root cause of suffering. Letting go allows us to live in greater harmony with inevitable change.

You may look at these attitudes and think we're asking you to change the way you are wholesale. In a sense, this is true. These attitudes are part of an antidote to a life that's out of balance; they point us toward the middle ground. Many of them are just the opposite of the way Western society teaches us to be, but you do have a choice in the matter. We remember one fellow in our class protesting quite earnestly, "But it's only an eight-week program!" True, but this can be the start of something that carries on for the rest of your life. Perhaps the best way to put these attitudes in context is to consider the opposite. You can be nonjudgmental and accepting, as we suggest, or imagine the opposite: someone who's a judgmental, impatient, know-it-all, paranoid control freak in denial of reality—your choice!

All kidding aside, though, sometimes these attitudes strike a negative chord for people living with cancer, because you may think we are suggesting that you just accept your diagnosis and prognosis passively, without trying to make things better. This is not at all the case; acceptance in the context of mindfulness is just about seeing things as they truly are. If you are dealing with cancer, there's no denying it. To accept something doesn't mean you have to like it or want it to be that way, but if it already *is* that way, what good does it do to close your eyes to it? How can you move on if you are unwilling to acknowledge the reality of the challenges you are facing?

Similarly, nonstriving doesn't mean you sit around in a funk all day on your meditation cushion; in fact we mentioned intention earlier, which may seem like a form of striving. Nonstriving is truly paradoxical, because the only way to actually achieve your intentions, once you have set them, is to then let them go to float in the background and, instead, put your efforts toward learning how to *be*, rather than *do* anything. You can see this clearly in the example of intending to relax: you can say to yourself, *I must relax—now!* and try really hard to do so, but we can pretty much guarantee that this approach won't work. The only way you will be able to relax is to truly let go of that intention, stop doing, and focus simply on learning to let things be. Sure, in the back of your mind, you still want to relax, but that may or may not happen. It's important that you learn to be okay with this. Anything less results in more struggle and works against your purpose. As you begin to meditate, accept whatever happens as just the way it is today.

Imagine a glass of silty or muddy water. The only way to purify the water is to allow it to sit still, and eventually the silt will settle to the bottom. Then the water becomes clear and palatable. You can't speed up the process by shaking the glass or trying to force the water to clear; that will just have the opposite effect. The same applies to relaxing your bodymind. So long as you are putting in the practice time with good faith, that's all you need to do.

SEEING THINGS ANEW

Let's now engage in a practice that's meant to call on the attitude of beginner's mind: seeing things as if for the first time, which also originally comes from Jon Kabat-Zinn (1990). As with all the practices to follow in this book, you can read the instructions in advance and then do the practice afterward, with or without the instructions, or go and get the raisins now and do the practice as you read it for the first time, stopping to lay down the book and take your time as you move through it. You could also ask someone to read the instructions aloud to you as you do the practice, or you could even make a recording of your own or someone else's voice to replay later. You could do this practice more than once or in different ways to notice how your experience changes each time.

PRACTICE 3.1
Mindfully Eating a Raisin

Take a raisin and place it in the palm of your hand. You are now going to experience it as if you have never seen this object before; in fact you have never seen *this* particular one. Take your time with this exploration; it can take several minutes or longer to complete. Now take the time to notice the object with all of your senses.

Beginning with sight, notice what shape it is, what color it is, what volume of space it fills up. Hold it with your thumb and forefinger and notice the way the light reflects off its surface as you roll it around, the nuance of color and light.

Now perhaps close your eyes and experience it with just the sense of touch in your hand. Can you sense its weight? Does it feel rough, smooth, sticky, hard, or soft? Can you feel the ridges in its surface? Are they uniform? Try manipulating it with your fingers and notice any changes in its shape or texture.

Slowly move it up to your nose and breathe in its scent. Does it have a smell? How would you characterize it? Is it sweet, earthy, salty, or musty, or does it have no smell at all? Is there any reaction in your body to the smell of the object? Check in with your mouth and your gut to see if your body is reacting. What thoughts are popping into your mind about the object? You may have memories of likes or dislikes or of times when you've interacted with objects like this in the past. They may be pleasant or unpleasant; just note whatever reactions you have, and then return to the sensory experience.

Now try holding it up to your ear; how does it baffle the sound entering your ear? Does it make any sound itself? Does it make a noise when you roll it around with your fingers? Do you feel silly listening to a raisin? Just take all of this in.

Now slowly move it to touch your lips; how is the sensation similar to or different from the touch on your hand and fingers? When you are ready, open your mouth and place it inside. Let it lie on your tongue for a moment; how does it feel? Is it smooth, rough, heavy, light? Notice how your tongue automatically knows how to move it around expertly. Note the urge to bite the object (or perhaps spit it out!).

When you are ready, bite down on the object, and note the burst of taste and the feeling of your teeth breaking through the skin. As you slowly chew the object, note the change in texture, the taste as it contacts different parts of your tongue, and the urge to swallow. When it's well chewed, allow yourself to swallow the object. Can you feel it moving down your esophagus toward your stomach? Note any residual flavor in your mouth. Is it possible to sense that you are now just one raisin heavier?

This practice highlights the attitude of beginner's mind, seeing something familiar as if for the first time. What was it like for you to eat a raisin in this way? How did it taste? Many people say it was the most delicious or flavorful raisin they ever had. How is it different from the way you usually eat such things? You may typically shovel them into your mouth in handfuls, barely stopping to chew. What if you ate the way you did in the practice more often? Would you eat less, perhaps enjoy your food more? We suggest you try to eat an entire meal in this way, stopping to lay down your utensils after you take a bite, maybe close your eyes, and chew each mouthful until it's done, noting texture and taste before picking up your utensils and moving on to the next bite. It may take longer, but we bet you will enjoy your meal much more by pausing to eat mindfully in this way.

PAYING ATTENTION TO BREATHING

The breath is an incredibly powerful tool and ally in the whole matter of meditation, stress reduction, and mindfulness. We often choose it as the focus of our mindfulness practice. One advantage of focusing on the breath is that it's always there; no matter where you are or what you are doing, so long as you are alive, you are breathing. Because of this, there's no barrier to practicing mindfulness of the breath at any time. The breath is always present, and perhaps because of this, most people rarely pay attention to it. It may seem a bit boring: in-out, in-out, and on and on. Actually, the breath is amazingly interesting when you stop to pay attention to it. Let's do that now. We don't want you to change your breathing in any way; just pay attention. Take a moment to try the following practice, "Mindful Breathing."

PRACTICE 3.2
Mindful Breathing

Take a seat that allows you to sit comfortably balanced and upright, with an erect back so that you are not slumping through the chest. Find a position that allows you to feel relaxed but alert. Now place one hand gently on your abdomen, just below your belly button (judgmental thoughts about needing to visit the gym more may arise; you can let those go now!). Place the other hand on your upper chest, just above your breastbone. Now close your eyes and pay attention to your breath. Don't try to control it in any way; just notice.

Perhaps note to yourself *in* as you breathe in, and *out* as you breathe out. Pay attention to any movement either hand senses as you breathe. Is one hand moving up and down more than the other? Where do you feel more movement? Is one or the other hand not moving at all? How long is the inbreath compared to the outbreath? Are they similar in length or different? Which is longer? Are there pauses or gaps after either the inbreaths or outbreaths? Does the breath flow smoothly, or is it jerky or broken in places?

Do you notice that the breath has changed at all now that you are paying attention to it? If it has, in what way did it change? Just sit quietly with the breath and notice if your mind wanders away to planning, worrying, or whatever other thoughts arise, and then draw your mind back to the breath when you notice this wandering. Can you become aware of other aspects of the body as you sit there, such as tension in the neck, shoulders, or arms, or perhaps your heart's beating or your stomach's grumbling? After a few minutes, allow your hands to fall to your sides, open your eyes, and return your attention to the room.

What did you notice from doing this practice? Often people find themselves trying to achieve a certain type of breathing because they have heard that one type is better than another, so the judgmental mind arises with thoughts like *My breathing is too shallow*, *My breath isn't long or deep enough*, and so on. The instruction was to not change the breath in any way; were you able to follow that directive? It's difficult, isn't it? Most people say that just the act of paying attention to the breath results in some changes, such as slowed breathing and increased feelings of relaxation. This isn't the case for everyone, though; some people find that paying attention to the breath makes it harder to breathe or makes them feel panicky. All of these experiences are common and nothing to worry about. Another common experience is that the mind wanders away from paying attention to the breath, often within seconds. Remember that paying attention is a skill that requires practice; if you keep it up, you will be able to focus for longer periods of time. Don't forget the little puppy, if you find yourself being harsh.

Diaphragmatic Breathing

Now, after telling you not to change or judge your breath, we are going to tell you about ways to breathe that are conducive to relaxation and focus. This is not to say that other ways of breathing are bad or wrong; they all just serve different purposes. The technique we use is variously called "diaphragmatic breathing," "abdominal breathing," "belly breathing," or simply "deep breathing." It's similar to what's known in yoga as the "complete breath." See figure 3.1 to better understand how the diaphragm muscle works when you breathe deeply.

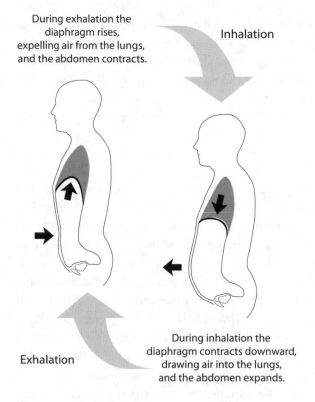

During exhalation the diaphragm rises, expelling air from the lungs, and the abdomen contracts.

Inhalation

During inhalation the diaphragm contracts downward, drawing air into the lungs, and the abdomen expands.

Exhalation

Figure 3.1 Diaphragmatic Breathing

The diaphragm is a sheet of muscle that transects the abdomen between the lungs and the abdominal organs. When you take a full breath, the diaphragm muscle flattens, pulling down and acting like a bellows that sucks air into the sacs of the lungs, where gases are exchanged. Carbon dioxide is expelled, and oxygen can be absorbed and circulated through the bloodstream as needed. As the diaphragm pulls down, the abdominal organs are squashed, hence the belly area rises up or expands. You can feel this movement with your hand. As you exhale, the diaphragm forces air out of the lungs by moving up, and the belly drops down.

When we conduct the mindful breathing practice, many people find that movement is primarily in the upper hand, hence the upper chest. This may be the result of learning to hold in our bellies so they don't expand as we breathe, or maintaining poor postural habits, which constrict breathing. If you breathe this way often, the consequence is that you can't expel breath fully out of your lungs or draw breath fully into your lungs. As a result, your breathing can be less efficient. With shallow breathing, air is partially exchanged with each breath, but old air that's full of carbon dioxide is not completely replaced with new, fresh air that's full of oxygen. An efficient exchange of these blood gases allows the body to function more optimally.

Oxygen is absorbed from the lung sacs into the bloodstream and carried to your muscles and organs, including your brain. In addition to nourishing your body, slow, deep breathing also has the effect of stimulating parts of your nervous system that allow you to relax and feel calm. We'll share more about this later. For now, we suggest using this type of breathing when you want to encourage a calm and alert state, such as when preparing for a period of meditation or while coordinating the breath and body during yoga practice. You might like to begin the next practice, the body scan, with a few slow, deep belly breaths, but you can practice this beneficial way of breathing anytime.

BODY SCAN

A fundamental practice, the body scan is the first formal meditation we do in the MBCR program. As you may have noticed when you did the breathing awareness practice earlier in this chapter, it can be hard to sustain your attention on the breath; the process is subtle, repetitive, and easy to drift away from.

The body scan practice adds other bodily sensations as objects of attention. Though some people find it easier to keep their attention on something solid, like a toe or an elbow, rather than the breath, the primary reason we begin mindfulness training with the body scan is to emphasize that all the meditation practices we will learn occur in the body; as we say, they are "embodied." Our society is very intellectual and often focused on thinking, the brain, and the head, but our bodies are where the action is. Every state of mind is reflected in a state of body, and our every emotion or thought has repercussions in the body. We will be discussing this a bit more in the next chapter.

Despite the body's central importance in our lives, it's easy to forget it. An oft-cited quote comes from the short story "A Painful Case," from James Joyce's *Dubliners* collection, about a character named Mr. Duffy. It was said, "He lived at a little distance from his body" (2000, 104). A similar observation might be made about many of us! As we go through life, it becomes easy to neglect our bodies. We can become so alienated from them that we may be unaware of how we are breathing or when our muscles are all tensed up. Illness itself can increase our sense of alienation from our bodies.

The body scan is a way of reacquainting ourselves with the body in a loving and gentle way. Especially if you have had cancer, you may feel that your body has betrayed you; you treated it as well as you could and still got cancer. You may be really angry at your body. You may also have had surgery or other treatments that caused your body to be very different now than it was before. Now is the time to start befriending again this body, the only one you will get in this life. Whatever its shortcomings, it has carried you this far. The body scan allows you to open up to the body, however it is, embracing it, flaws and all. Note that in the instructions, as in several meditations throughout this book, we have included dashes to indicate that you should rest for a breath or two before moving on to the next phrase. If done in this manner, the practice will take you thirty to forty-five minutes, but you can also do it more quickly. Additionally, as in other practices in this book, we have used a suggestive, rather than directive, form of instruction to reflect a process that's unfolding, and we have minimized the use of pronouns (such as "you" and "your") to emphasize awareness over personal agency. We suggest making a recording of these body scan instructions, so you can listen to them whenever you like. With practice, you will be able to do a self-directed body scan without instruction.

PRACTICE 3.3
Body Scan

The body scan invites you to enter and dwell in a deep state of relaxation and awareness, a kind of wakeful sleep. Remember, as you relax deeply, you assume an active and powerful role in supporting the healing powers of your bodymind.

Choose a comfortable place to lie down, where you can rest peacefully, perhaps a mat or rug on the floor, a bed, or a reclining chair. For comfort you may wish to support parts of your body with cushions or pillows.

Lying now—facing upward—resting on the back—in this place of comfort and ease—perhaps allowing the eyes to gently close— beginning to sense the surrendering of the bodymind to the firm support of the earth or floor beneath—perhaps adjusting the body to its full length, chest open—arms resting beside—palms open and up—legs comfortably apart—allowing the feet to fall open to the sides by their own weight—finding a position that's comfortable.

Lying in stillness—now—for a while—except for the flow of breath and energy and awareness—letting go of any tendency to want things to be any different than they are—allowing things to be exactly—exactly as they are.

Following along as much as possible, noticing bodily sensations—feelings—any activity of the mind along the way—noticing and letting go of any judgmental or critical thoughts—opening awareness to whatever the bodymind encounters—remembering that there's no right or wrong way to feel—that feelings are feelings—simply accepting and allowing whatever feelings arise—knowing that it's okay.

Now shifting awareness gently to attend to the breath—the ebbing and flowing breath within—following its natural, easy rhythm—just as it is—simply experiencing the sensation—as the air moves in—and out—of being—perhaps noticing—with the internal sense of awareness—the rhythmic movement of ribs and belly—the rising—falling—falling—rising—of each outbreath—perhaps noting the feeling of letting go as the bodymind—releases—and cool air moves in—and warm, moist air—moves out—out—and—in.

Now shifting awareness gently to the right foot and lower leg, perhaps beginning with the toes—feeling each toe individually and the spaces between them—becoming aware of whatever sensations reveal themselves in this part of the body—such as tingling— warmth—or coolness, a sense of the size or shape—maybe little or no sensation—and that's all right too—whatever is there— noticing it all—and letting it go as you shift awareness to the next perception—and the next—awareness of the foot—heel—arch— Achilles tendon—the calf—and shin—all the way to the knee—the back of the knee—sides—and front—now, with the next breath in—allowing the whole lower leg and foot to fill with awareness— noticing its presence and energy—breathing out, allowing the lower leg to dissolve in awareness—effervescent.

And now shifting awareness to the upper leg—thigh—hip— front and back—again, just noticing—feeling—accepting—letting go and moving on—noticing whatever can be noticed, sensed, felt— letting awareness explore any and all that presents itself—feelings, thoughts that arise—memories—whatever comes—experiencing it—in awareness—and letting it go.

Now, with the next inbreath, sensing the leg as a whole— filling it with awareness—at its periphery and its core—from the toes to the hip—and then with the outbreath, letting it all go.

Dissolving in awareness as attention now shifts to the left foot and leg—taking however much time it takes—aware of any and every perception on this side—guiding awareness through—toes—each toe—each surface—foot inside and out—top and bottom—sensing bones and flesh—shape and energy—the leg—and so on—now, with the next breath in, allowing awareness to apprehend the whole leg—sensing it all—and now releasing, dissolving and shifting awareness once again.

Now to the pelvis—noticing any tension or holding on—allowing that awareness to initiate letting go—releasing any holding, any tension—now exploring the pelvic region—from the pelvic floor—the genitals—the buttocks—hips—up to the *waist—with each breath, releasing any holding on or clenching—in these sensitive and vulnerable parts—aware of the capacity for opening and closing to the environment—allowing—letting go—in the safety of this moment—continuing to sense and be aware of whatever is encountered here—perhaps an awareness of the movement or pressure changes that occur with each breath—whatever is encountered, feeling—thoughts—noticing—and moving on—now, with the next breath in—filling this whole region with awareness, and with the outbreath—allowing the pelvis to dissolve in awareness.*

Shifting now—to the torso—the belly—sides—back—lower and upper—the breast—chest—ribs—shoulders—arms—hands—fingers—sensing—noticing—aware of what's here—exploring with awareness—with curiosity—perhaps a sense of the breadth of the torso—the shape of its outline—contours—its surface—the skin—its depth—the core—and noticing the breath again, moving in and out—expanding subtly and contracting over and over—next—breathing in—letting awareness fill the whole torso—now breathing out—dissolving and shifting.

Letting awareness move now to the neck—throat—face—scalp—ears—the space between the ears—eyes—nose—mouth—softening and releasing any tension—letting the jaw be easy—the tongue go soft in the mouth.

Now—with the next breath in—sensing or envisioning drawing energy or awareness in through the top of the head—perhaps through a blowhole, like a whale or dolphin—and awareness sweeping down—coursing through the body, filling it up and sweeping it clear—energizing—purifying—enlightening—with energy—letting the energy sweep down and leave the body through the soles of the feet while releasing the breath outward—becoming a channel of energy—sweeping in—swirling—filling and now emptying—with each breath cycle—and now easily—letting go—resting in awareness—awareness of the whole of being—at once—appreciating completeness—the wonder of it all—just the way it is—a miracle of being—resting quietly now for a few moments, letting go—content to be just as you are—letting go—into stillness and awareness.

After a few minutes, rouse yourself gently. As you go about the rest of your day—your living—perhaps you can carry with you a lingering peacefulness and sense of comfort, qualities that are available to you whenever you can remember—to stop—pause—let go—and dwell in awareness.

___

Notice how you feel after a body scan. Though there's no correct way to feel, often people have a sense of quiet relaxation and focus. It's also not uncommon for people to find that they drift off to sleep, because this meditation can be a deeply relaxing experience. The intention of the practice, however, is more akin to "falling awake" than falling asleep: although you may feel relaxed, you are also very alert. If you find yourself drifting to sleep, you can try practicing at a different time of day (before a meal rather than afterward, or first thing in the morning), sitting up, or keeping your eyes open rather than closed. At times you may become aware that your attention has drifted away, and you can then choose to refocus, beginning anew or resuming at the point you last recall.

Sometimes people also find that the body scan increases their anxiety or puts emphasis on body issues they would rather not deal with. For example, Sarah, a fifty-five-year-old married breast-cancer survivor, found her anxiety building as she worked up to the breast area the first time she did a body scan. She'd had surgery to remove the lump from one breast two months earlier, and there was a scar that felt tight and pulled when she raised her arm: she thought it was extremely ugly, kind of purple and puckered. She had avoided showing it to her husband and tried not to even look at it herself. As the group instructor guiding the meditation moved toward this area, Sarah could feel her body tensing and her anxiety building. When she got there, she tried to follow the instructions and pay attention to her bodily sensations and feelings. She tried to keep breathing steadily, but found tears leaking out the sides of her eyes, and sobbed quietly.

She felt such a loss and sadness for the way her body used to be, how much she'd been through, and how she would never be the same. For her, this was the beginning of a healing process. Day after day, each time she did the body scan, it got easier for her to pay attention to her misshapen breast, until eventually her grief subsided, and she felt something more like gentle kindness toward all that her body had endured.

HOW TO PRACTICE THESE SKILLS

This is a lot to learn at first; we recommend beginning by setting aside a specific time each day for practicing the body scan; usually about thirty minutes is good. Then, each day try to work through the instructions, purposefully applying the attitudes of nonjudgment and acceptance to your experience. You may also begin to pay more attention to what and how you eat, aiming to eat perhaps one meal each day with awareness, free of the distractions of TV, radio, newspaper, and so on. This is another way to care for your body. You can begin to use diaphragmatic breathing anytime during the day that you notice yourself feeling tense or riled up; purposefully move your breath down into your belly area, slowing and smoothing out the flow of breath. Practice for at least a week or two before moving on to the sitting meditation described in the next chapter.

CHAPTER 4

Responding to Stress

In chapter 2 we talked about the stress response and described the typical experience of stress in your body. We asked you to think about your habitual patterns of reacting to stress and to begin using these symptoms as cues for practicing some of the tools for stress reduction we outlined in chapter 3, such as diaphragmatic breathing. In this chapter we draw a clearer distinction between your typical stress *reaction*—the habitual reflexive behaviors you may automatically experience during an episode you consider stressful—and the more purposive stress *response*—your considered and careful response to the stressors that present themselves to you. As you will see, this distinction can be very helpful as you move through your daily life, encountering those small everyday hassles and larger challenges.

REACTING VS. RESPONDING TO STRESS

We include figures 4.1 and 4.2 to show you the differences between a typical stress reaction and the more purposive stress response you will learn through this program. These figures are adapted from Jon Kabat-Zinn's book *Full Catastrophe Living*, chapter 19 (Kabat-Zinn 1990).

The Stress Reaction

In figure 4.1, "Reacting to Stress," at the top of the picture are external stress events. Now this can be anything from running late for an appointment to receiving a cancer diagnosis, from long-term events like serving as caregiver for an elderly parent to discrete events like filing your income tax at the last minute before the deadline. The key thing about external stress events is that they are not stressful *in and of themselves*; it's the next step, your appraisal of their significance, that determines whether you perceive external events as stressful. Your perception also determines your bodily reaction to the events.

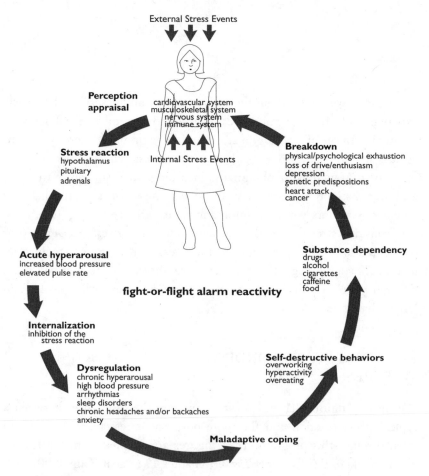

Figure 4.1 Reacting to Stress

This process of perception and appraisal happens quickly and automatically; often you may not even be aware that it's happening. Of course, running late is stressful; you think, *People are waiting for me!* But not everyone finds similar situations to be this stressful. Someone else might think, *Oh well, I'll just give them a call and let them know I'm running late—no worries!* Of course, nearly everyone who receives a cancer diagnosis finds it stressful, but not every person experiences even that event in the same way. Someone who considers cancer to be a certain death sentence unquestionably reacts differently than does someone who knows that overall survival rates for many types of cancer are higher than 90 percent. We will talk more about our interpretations of events and the stories we tell ourselves in chapter 7; for now, suffice it to say that this step of appraisal is an important one for determining the rest of the cycle.

THE PHYSICAL REACTION

Once you have decided, consciously or unconsciously, how stressful an event is, your body kicks in with a proportionate stress reaction. Remember the fight-or-flight reaction we described in chapter 2? Here is where it would be triggered. As shown in figure 4.1, your cardiovascular, nervous, muscular, and immune systems all kick in, causing you to experience symptoms such as a racing heart, increased blood pressure, sweaty palms, and muscle tension. Your body prepares to face the threat head on, or if that strategy won't likely be safe or successful, you get ready to run for the hills as fast as your legs can carry you. Hence, the blood flows into your arms and legs, your heart beats faster to get it there, and your blood pressure goes up. At the same time, blood is diverted away from your digestive system, since that type of housekeeping can generally wait until the acute threat has passed. Then it's time to get back to the day-to-day chores of eating, digesting, and resting. This system works well if the stressors you encounter are all of the very acute, time-limited variety.

But what if that perceived threat never passes? What if the stress you experience is generated from a thought in your head rather than an actual threat in the environment? If we consider a stressor like living with cancer, caring for an elderly relative, or having chronic worry, the stressor may not go away for months or even years. So what do many people do to cope? A first line of defense may be to just push it away, minimize it, repress it, or deny the extent of the problem: *Yeah, sure, it's difficult, but I feel fine.* This is what's called "internalization" in figure 4.1. Unfortunately, internalizing just drives the disturbance out of our conscious awareness, but the distressing situation is not fundamentally resolved and is easily reawakened. Internalization of stress may remove the triggering events from center stage in our thoughts, yet they continue to affect our physiology, the way we feel, and our behavior.

If not counterbalanced, the physical reactions to everyday stress can become chronic and more pronounced. You may start to experience *dysregulation*, a loss of balance, in a number of physical systems, which can result in persistently elevated blood pressure, heart abnormalities like an arrhythmic heartbeat, and other damaging effects on the body. High levels of activation and disturbance of the body's self-regulating mechanisms can result in a cascade of difficulties. Difficulty calming down enough to sleep properly at night can compound the problems. In addition, for many, prolonged muscle tension can result in headaches, backaches, and other bodily pain and discomfort.

THE BEHAVIORAL REACTION

Once your body is in overdrive like this and you begin suffering the consequences of prolonged hyperarousal, you may be willing do pretty much anything to just get a good night's rest or feel relaxed. Often at this point, people turn to the old standbys: alcohol, cigarettes, sleeping pills, or even comfort foods like ice cream or potato chips. Going shopping is the temporary salve for many. Who can really blame you if you find yourself falling for one of these coping methods on occasion? They're easy, legal, easily accessible, quite commonly used, and accepted by society, plus they seem to help a bit.

Others who want to avoid these substances or activities may bury their troubles in chronic overwork or excessive busyness. In fact, some of these behaviors, such as workaholism, are often praised and can lead to financial and career rewards. In fact, if you're not always so busy or constantly on the run, some people might question whether you're doing enough with your life. But denying the problem and covering it up with substances or distractions doesn't address the root problem or the persistent physical reactions in your body.

THE CONSEQUENCES

All of these behaviors are really quick fixes, short-term solutions that have a real downside. If you look at figure 4.1 again, the last arrow leads to a breakdown of the system. There's only so much strain and stress your body can take before something has to give. How this happens largely depends on your genetic makeup and any predispositions or vulnerabilities you already have. Some people are at risk for developing heart disease or addictions; others may be more susceptible to depression. Anyone may feel simply exhausted and unable to sustain the quick pace of life. Many people with cancer turn to stress reduction, because they have come to believe that the impact of stress on their immune systems made them vulnerable to cancer. Some suspect that their unhealthy coping behaviors were a factor in their developing the disease.

As we discussed in chapter 2, the belief that there's a direct cause-and-effect relationship between stress and cancer is a controversial one. We know that some unhealthy lifestyle factors adopted under the sway of chronic stress (such as smoking and drinking) can contribute to cancer's development, but there are many other causal factors. We think it's safe to say that most people would like to do everything they can to improve their chances of remaining cancer-free in the future. No one can guarantee that improving your resilience and modifying your stress response will move you to that goal, but we do know that it certainly won't hurt and that you'll be much happier and enjoy life more in the bargain! The next section presents an alternative to this downwardly spiraling stress reaction.

The Stress Response

Before you get too discouraged about the cycle shown in figure 4.1, let us show you the alternative, which we refer to as the *stress response*. It may seem a bit overwhelming to find yourself on that downwardly spiraling cycle of maladaptive stress reaction, but there are many avenues or detours you can take to get off that pathway. In fact, at every juncture in the previous figure, there's a corresponding exit ramp that we will describe for you.

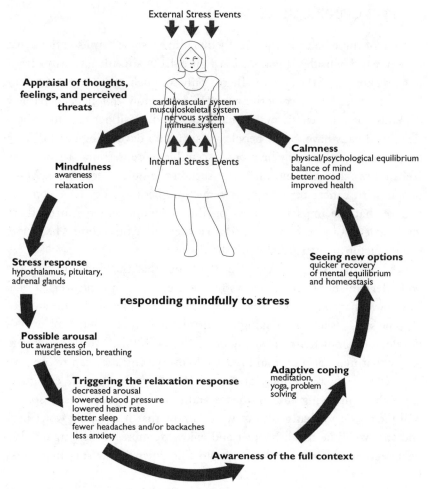

Figure 4.2 Responding to Stress

In figure 4.2 we still begin with external stress events, which are not going to go away; there will always be traffic, demanding jobs, health concerns, and people to care for. However, the first step, your perception or appraisal of the situation, can benefit from applying some mindful awareness. Just noticing that you have a decision point here can be a breakthrough, especially since our patterns of thought often become so ingrained that they're automatic. You can stop and say to yourself, *Well,*

I have a choice here: I can interpret this as a catastrophe, or I can decide that this is something I can handle.

There may still be an initial surge of arousal even if you decide the stressor is something you can handle, but it may be more transitory and less pronounced than if you decided it was a full-blown catastrophe. In addition to the physical and mental arousal, you can also hold an awareness of this arousal and eventually apply different coping techniques. Rather than head for the bar, the refrigerator, or your computer to bury yourself in distractions, you can calm yourself with a few deep breaths and sit with your thoughts for a moment, or call a friend to share your feelings. You may be able to see options you hadn't considered. By applying a variety of techniques, you may be able to diminish your stress response and find a place of calm equilibrium. Eventually, with practice, you can learn to go through this process quite quickly and more often.

How to Become Less Reactive and More Responsive to Stress

Don't worry if you still find yourself swept away by your reactions to stress. The first step is to begin to notice when this happens, and *immediately* apply some mindfulness techniques. You may not notice your reactions until you find yourself yelling and spitting curses at the driver who cut you off. That's okay. Take a moment at that point to pull over, shut your eyes, and just breathe deeply. Notice how your body feels: can you feel your heart racing, your palms sweating, your body shaking all over in anger? Stay with it. Does it change as you focus on the sensations? Can you allow your muscles to relax and your heart to slow down?

After the physical reaction has subsided, ask yourself, *Why did I get so upset? It wasn't my fault; the other driver was being rude and inconsiderate, and I have a lot on my mind and many things to get done today. Could I have reacted differently? Who is the one who suffered most from my outburst?* The other person may have been shocked and embarrassed, but you subjected yourself to the miserable experience of feeling angry and stressing your bodily systems. You could have simply brushed it off and carried on. One of our patients shared with us the thought that anger is like a poison you give to yourself but expect somebody else to die from. By reacting so severely, you give someone else a tremendous amount of power over how you feel; do you really want to relinquish that power?

59

It might take a long time of practicing in this way—reacting and then taking stock of why you reacted so strongly and how you felt during the course of it—but eventually you may be able to notice more and more quickly the buildup to a full-blown stress reaction, and stop it in its tracks, if that's the appropriate thing to do. Of course, stopping to breathe deeply as a speeding train bears down on you wouldn't do; there are circumstances where the stress reaction is useful, but if it's not a situation where fighting or running makes sense, it's probably better to learn to head it off at the pass. Mindfulness provides the access point to bring healing responses into the equation.

In fact, in our studies with breast-cancer and prostate-cancer patients who had finished their primary treatments, we monitored stress-response measures including production of the stress hormone cortisol (Carlson et al. 2004) and the immune system's inflammatory cytokines (Carlson et al. 2003). We found that after the program and up to twelve months later, production of these substances had decreased substantially in the MBCR participants (Carlson et al. 2007). We don't know precisely what this means in terms of disease outcomes, but it does suggest that the participants were better able to modulate stress in their lives.

FORMAL AND INFORMAL MINDFULNESS PRACTICES

In the last chapter we introduced mindful attitudes as well as the more formal practice of the body scan. Next we will introduce another formal practice, sitting meditation. But first, we think it's important that you become aware of the distinction between what we call "formal" and "informal" mindfulness or meditation practices. Formal meditation is when you set aside a time, assume a specific position, and say to yourself, *Now I am going to meditate*; this corresponds with the little-m mindfulness we introduced in chapter 3.

This type of practice is very important, because it will teach you discipline and ensure that you put in the time required to learn this new skill. Just as with learning any other skill, such as playing the piano or playing tennis, you are not a virtuoso overnight. It takes many hours of playing scales and returning serves to reach even a basic level of competence. Similarly, with meditation it can take weeks or months of practice before you can sustain some measure of present-moment awareness over a significant period of time. In effect you need to train your mind. Formal practice helps you get there.

But what good is it if you are mindful and aware on your cushion, but at no other time during your day; if you are kind and accepting when you meditate, but cruel and judgmental with your family and friends? This is where the informal practice, or big-M mindfulness, comes in. Informal mindfulness is the practice of remembering to apply your awareness and mindful attitudes at any time. You can always stop and tune in to your breath; notice your bodily sensations; and choose to slow down, take a few breaths, relax your muscles, quit daydreaming, and engage in your activities with full awareness, an open heart, and acceptance.

How often do you miss opportunities to be kind, to listen with full awareness, to be patient instead of rushed and frazzled? These opportunities are always present, and your informal mindfulness practice is to start bringing more awareness to your everyday activities and applying some of the mindful attitudes, such as slowing down and accepting yourself, others, and situations as they are. When you are in a frustrating situation you can't change, try just saying to yourself, *It is what it is.* That's certainly true; it is what it is, and you can either rail against it and make yourself miserable and wound up, or just accept that it is indeed exactly what it is. And by the way, it's also constantly changing, so don't get too used to it!

Formal and informal practices complement each other perfectly; you can't really have a complete mindfulness practice without both approaches. In formal practice you have a chance to sit with uncomfortable emotions that may arise and deal with them in a different way than in the frenzy of everyday life. You can choose to hold impatience in your awareness, for example, rather than push and pull to make things happen your way. The formal practice is a microcosm for your everyday life, so all the things that challenge you in life will also eventually arise to challenge you in meditation practice. This is great! Don't be frustrated when your mind brings up those old patterns; instead say, *Wonderful! Welcome impatience! Welcome sadness! Now's my chance to practice being with you and just seeing what you are all about, without having to rush to make you go away.* Surprisingly, you may find that the impatience, the sadness, or whatever demon you're encountering passes or transforms without your having to do anything about it at all, other than accept it just as it is.

So this relearning or training in formal practice can give you new ideas and confidence for your informal encounters in everyday life. You may think to yourself, *I notice I am really angry now and want to yell at someone, but in meditation yesterday it was okay to feel angry, and eventually the feeling faded away on its own; maybe if I just breathe a bit now instead of yelling, it will be okay.* You may be surprised at the outcome.

SITTING MEDITATION

Many people consider sitting meditation to be the heart of the formal practice, so they do it almost exclusively. Of course, sitting is just the posture, and what goes on in your mind varies considerably. Here we will introduce you to basic mindful awareness in the sitting posture. We typically begin with awareness of the breath and expand over time to include awareness of other senses, feelings, and thoughts.

Sitting Posture

Let's begin with the basic posture. First of all, you don't have to sit wrapped up like a pretzel on the floor to meditate. You can sit in a straight-backed chair, on a meditation stool, or on the floor with a cushion. It often works well to sit on a yoga mat that's folded in half, or on a soft quilt or carpet to be sure your knees and ankles have sufficient padding, and then slip a cushion under the back of your buttocks for some height. If possible, your legs will cross and your knees will rest on the floor so that your knees and tailbone make a triangular shape. If your knees are up in the air when you sit cross-legged, it's a good idea to support them with folded blankets or pillows underneath to avoid too much strain. If you are on a chair, try moving toward the front edge, or conversely, wedge your hips right to the back of the chair. You want to be sitting upright instead of slumping against the chair. Plant both feet firmly on the floor at a distance that allows the knees to be level with or lower than the hips.

In either case you can rest your hands on your knees or in your lap, with your palms facing up or down; notice the different feel each position engenders. Notice the two bony sit bones at the very base of the pelvis; they should rest on your cushion or the chair, with your pelvis tilted just slightly forward. This will maintain the curve in the lower lumbar spine so that your back isn't rounded and slumped over. This position also helps to keep your chest open. Ensuring that your sit bones are at least as high as your knees is key. Allow your shoulder blades to move back and slide down your spine so that your shoulders are relaxed and farther away from your ears. Try to maintain this posture throughout the sitting meditation as much as possible, but without too much strain. Feel free to make adjustments if you experience pain, but avoid moving mindlessly from restlessness or fidgeting.

Practicing Sitting Meditation

These instructions will probably help the most if you make a recording of them beforehand or have someone else read them to you as you meditate. Alternatively, you could read a paragraph and practice for a few minutes before moving on to read and practice the next section. You can also order CDs of these meditations from our website: www. mindfulnesscalgary.ca.

PRACTICE 4.1
Sitting Meditation

Find a comfortable sitting position where your spine is upright, your head is gently balanced on the stalk of your neck, and your shoulders are drawn back and sliding down the spine. If you are seated in a chair, move forward to the edge and place your feet flat on the floor, or rest them on a cushion or riser. Make sure your spine is balanced and not leaning into the chair back, if possible. If you are seated on a cushion, make sure your hips are elevated so that your legs are resting or supported with cushions to avoid strain. Rest your hands on your knees or in your lap, one on top of the other. Settle into a position where you can remain comfortable and still for some time.

Now allowing focus to come to the inflow and outflow of breath— with the mind relaxed and spacious—without having to create anything—simply feeling the gentle rising of the belly, the abdomen, with each inbreath—and the falling with each outbreath—allowing the breath to be natural—noting its inflow and outflow, without trying to force or control it in any way—noting each in and out, each rising and falling, and allowing a settling into the breath's even rhythm—allowing the mind to rest in that place—feeling the movement of the breath.

While feeling the breath, making a mental note to sharpen concentration—noting in *while feeling the breath go in—and* out *while feeling it leave—or saying* rising *and* falling *with the sensations in the chest or belly—very gently, very quietly in the mind—just supporting the awareness of the actual sensations—just noting* in *and* out, rising *and* falling*—bringing the mind back to the breath time and again.*

Never needing to make the breath special—each breath being unique in itself and not necessarily deep or long, or different from however it is and however it changes—because it's happening anyway, simply being aware of it—one breath at a time.

Possibly noticing attention wandering—this is okay—perhaps getting lost in thought, planning, remembering, or worrying— perhaps not consciously having noticed breath for quite some time— no problem—no need to judge or analyze, or try to figure out how it slipped away—no matter—just gently letting go of the distraction and beginning again—letting go and returning attention to the breath's easy inflow and outflow.

Beginning again and again—the essential art of the practice— over and over, beginning anew with patience and equanimity.

While sitting and feeling the breath, possibly noticing sensations arising in the body that are strong enough to draw attention from the breath—this is okay—if this happens, not needing to struggle or push the sensation away—just letting awareness settle fully on the experience of the sensation—perhaps becoming the new object of meditation—with the breath still an anchor in the background.

As strong sensations arise, making a quiet mental note of the experience in this moment—pain, itching, tingling, pressure— whatever word emerges to describe the sensation—but without judging as good or bad, right or wrong—just allowing the self to be with the changing nature of the sensation, without holding onto the sensation or tensing around it—the same quality of awareness as with breath—spacious, open, relaxed, free—without trying to change or control the sensations—noting that they change on their own—and just relaxing around the experience of discomfort—not needing to fight or struggle with sensation.

In the face of an unpleasant experience, possibly wishing to push it away, or perhaps feeling angry or fearful about it—perhaps feeling mental and physical tension in relation to the sensation or discomfort—simply noting this reaction and returning to the direct experience—relaxing around the shifting sensations.

If fighting against the pain—hating it or growing tenser— choosing to shift or change posture—doing so with intention— thinking about where to move each part of the body—shifting mindfully and beginning again in stillness and ease—noting the shift of sensations while settling.

Just returning to the breath—feeling the beginning of this very breath and the end of it—the beginning of the rising movement and the end—the beginning of the outbreath and the end—the beginning of the falling of the belly and the end—remaining present with each breath as if it were the first and last—applying this immediacy of attention—simply being here with nowhere to go, nothing to do— simply being here—this is life—right in this moment—in this one breath—in and out.

Now allowing focus to broaden somewhat from the pinpoint of the breath—to expand to include other types of awareness— while maintaining that contact with the breath as the anchor and returning if attention is drawn away into the past or future— allowing focus to move to awareness of sound—simply hearing— noting the effortless quality of hearing—not needing to make anything happen—sound happening all by itself—simply hearing sounds within the body—sounds in the room—sounds of other people—sounds of the room itself—sounds outside the room—a certain quality of silence—not needing to make sounds come or go—not needing to identify or label sounds, to judge as good or bad, pleasant or not—hearing without effort—with awareness—the sound appearing—hearing it—connecting with it—letting it fade away—remaining present to the soundscape.

Allowing awareness to expand now to include feelings and emotions—noting the emotional tone in the mind—calm, peaceful, bored?—happiness, restlessness, sadness, fear, neutrality?—opening to and recognizing the emotional background just as with the breath, physical sensation, or sound—being aware of any prominent emotions arising—noting them in the body—in the belly, the heart, the throat, behind the eyes—noting emotions as they inhabit the body—accepting each emotion and seeing it as it rises and falls, shifts and changes with each passing breath—neither right nor wrong—just allowing it to appear and disappear.

Opening now to thoughts in the mind—without thinking thoughts—just watching them rise and fall—asking What will the next thought be?*—detecting the very beginning—the seed of thought in the mind—seeing its rising, peaking, falling—its floating like a cloud across the vast expanse of clear, blue sky—seeing the thoughts coming and going as fleeting mind moments—seeing them come and go, whether they are willed or not—thoughts without a thinker—not needing to get wrapped up in their content—despite possibly distressing thoughts, allowing awareness of thinking to remain balanced—awareness remaining calm, peaceful, accepting things as they are—knowing you are not your thoughts—knowing you are much more than these fleeting mind moments.*

Finally, coming to the breath again—simply feeling the stretching, pressure, and movement of the chest and abdomen as the breath comes and goes—in and out—nothing to do—just being with the breath—aware of each inflow and outflow—even as distractions arise—plans and images and aches and pains—all are okay—noting when contact is lost and simply returning again and again—the heart of the practice—beginning again and again—returning with patience and gentleness.

Ending the session with gently opening eyes—taking a few moments to listen to whatever sounds are present—feeling the body—seeing if some of this quality of presence and connection can be brought forward as you move out into the world.

Practice Times

This sitting meditation should take about thirty minutes if you read it slowly, pausing between sections. We recommend starting sitting meditation with shorter, say ten- or twenty-minute, sessions, but soon working up to a full thirty-minute session. If you have practiced the body scan for a week or so, now would be a good time to start alternating between it and sitting meditation every other day.

CHAPTER 5

Mindful Movement

Applying mindful awareness to practicing any of a number of movement disciplines, such as yoga, tai chi, or dance, is an excellent way to engage in self-care while developing greater harmony and wisdom within your evolving mind-body relationship.

Because we think it provides an especially useful path to support your recovery process, yoga is an integral part of our approach. Yoga can help to restore and expand functional capabilities your treatment may have affected. Yoga also provides a gentle and compassionate way to nurture yourself while bringing some joy into your process of reacquainting with yourself as a living, moving, and embodied being. Numerous health benefits traditionally ascribed to yoga have found scientific support in recent times, including improved flexibility, balance, and endurance.

Many people in our program have felt that they were too old, inflexible, or disabled from their cancer treatments to even get down on the floor, let alone practice unfamiliar and unusual movements. If you feel that way too, don't be intimidated by the word "yoga"; we won't ask you to stand on your head or wrap your leg around your neck! The movement practice we will describe is fundamentally about becoming more aware of your physical body. It doesn't matter at all how "perfectly" you can do the movements; please do whatever you can and make sensible modifications, if necessary, along the way. Remember to adopt beginner's mind, approaching this as an adventure, with a sense of discovery and wonder.

We recall a number of people who were reluctant to try yoga. One woman in particular was self-conscious about her weight, and she worried that she might not be able to get up off the floor once she was down there. We encouraged her to give it a try, and she surprised herself with her ability to do most of the lying postures with little difficulty, although her breathing was heavy and her wrists felt a bit sore when supporting her weight in the poses on hands and knees. She managed to get up by leaning on a chair, and she carried on with the practice at home each day. By the end of eight weeks, she marveled at how much stronger her joints felt, how her breathing was less and less labored, and how much easier the poses had become.

In this chapter we will provide some practical guidance for developing a yoga practice along the lines of what we teach in the MBCR program. You will find these instructions useful, whether you are practicing on your own at home or as part of a group in a class or yoga studio. As with learning any new skill, it helps to have the guidance of an experienced teacher along the way. However, using the following information will help you to build a solid foundation for a personal yoga practice you can take with you wherever you go.

If you already practice yoga or have done so in the past, we encourage you to rededicate yourself with renewed enthusiasm. Beginning each yoga session by clarifying your intention to honor your body and maintain a mindful quality of attention throughout the session may refresh aspects of your practice that have grown stale. A dose of beginner's mind can help you to avoid drudgery and to inject a sense of playful discovery into your practice.

THE CONTEXT OF YOGA

Yoga is, first and foremost, an ancient spiritual tradition. The ultimate origins of yoga are lost in the mists of time, but the Vedic scriptures of India in the second millennium BCE documented the use of the term to describe an approach for disciplining the mind for spiritual development (Feuerstein 2000, 342). *Yoga* is often translated from the original Sanskrit as "union," suggesting the uniting of mind, body, and spirit. The root of the word means to "yoke" or "harness," which conveys the sense of yoga as a discipline.

From its ancient roots, yoga evolved to become prominent as one of six orthodox systems of Indian philosophy and, sometime in the second century BCE, was codified in the Yoga Sutras of Patanjali, who was a sage. Though classical yoga encompasses a range of ethical and meditative practices, we will focus on the disciplined use of physical postures (*asanas*) and, to a lesser extent, breath control (*pranayama*), which is an integral part of asana practice.

FOUNDATIONS FOR YOGA PRACTICE

Following some basic guidelines will set you off on the right foot (pun intended).

Safety

It's sensible to warm up and loosen the body at the start of your yoga session. This could be as simple as moving your limbs through their range of motion with gentle swings, slowly rotating your joints, or improvising a small dance. Yoga is traditionally done barefoot. If you wear socks or some light footwear, it's important that your feet be free to move and that you have good traction with the ground or floor. Take care to have a flat surface. Yoga mats help on both counts and are widely available. Mats come in various thicknesses. Be aware that though a thicker mat provides more cushioning for bones, it may feel less stable, and it may even snag or twist a toe as you move.

Move in and out of yoga asanas gradually and sensitively. There's a bit of an art to finding that point within an asana that's just at the edge of what's comfortable. From that point, using the breath, gravity, stabilizing or agonist (opposing) muscle contraction, and patience gently encourages the muscles to release and the connective tissues to lengthen, allowing the body's energy to flow freely. As best you can, sustain awareness of bodily sensations and the breath moment by moment. Inability to keep the breath smooth and regular is a signal to reduce the intensity of your effort to the point where you can restore rhythmic breathing.

Especially for beginners, never rush or throw yourself aggressively into poses. Take care to maintain good alignment in your joints. There should be a sense of maintaining space in the joints and a feeling of uplift throughout the body in standing postures, without stiffness or rigidity. Know and respect your vulnerabilities. If you have had injuries or recent surgery, you may have to reduce the range of motion of certain poses, modify them, use straps or bolsters for support, or avoid those poses altogether. If an instructor is available, relate your concerns and ask for guidance. Talk to your physician and discuss any health concerns before undertaking yoga practice.

Progression

Start with simple postures and progress to more challenging ones. Many classic yoga poses are basic in the sense of being foundational. They have stood the test of time and are no less important than advanced poses. Think of basic asanas as the main course, while fancier variations can serve as dessert. Just as a ballet dancer never stops practicing pliés and a musician never stops going through scales, the basic poses remain valuable regardless of how proficient you become.

Breath and Movement

A natural coordination occurs between breath and movement in that each movement is associated with an inbreath or outbreath. Typically when the body is contracted, folded, or twisted, you exhale; and when you expand, open, or extend the body, you inhale. If you are unsure, a little experimentation to determine which pattern of breath most supports the movement will likely clear things up. Breathing through the nose, if possible, is standard for yoga. For some asanas that involve bending to the side, a bit of breath can be retained before the bottom of the breath is reached to provide support and stability to the spine.

Yoga Sequences

Yoga asanas are often linked together in sequences designed to complement and balance the effects of the poses, and unify them into a logical whole that can flow from one pose to another. In this chapter we have included illustrations and instructions for two basic sequences, one you do while lying on your mat and one you do standing, that you will likely find within your capability even as a beginner. Before long, you might find it fun to learn other traditional sequences in a yoga class or by piecing together several poses to create a customized sequence of your own.

Dynamic vs. Sustained

You can do yoga asanas and flowing sequences of several asanas in either a dynamic way or one that's static or sustained. In dynamic practice, each movement is repeated in a rhythmic way several times, typically with one inbreath and outbreath per repetition, or movement flows from one asana directly into another. Alternatively, you could sustain any pose or each of a series of poses for a longer period of time. Sustaining a pose for the length of five or six complete breaths allows the body to accommodate to the pose so that reflexes, which protect tissues from sudden stresses by limiting the range of motion, release. Usually, dynamic practice precedes and prepares the body suitably for sustaining poses.

GETTING STARTED

Look over the figures that follow to get an overall sense of the logic and flow of the asanas. If you are a yoga beginner you may need to consult the figures periodically until you learn the sequences and can link them together smoothly. We suggest you begin with dynamic practice, repeating each of the movements rhythmically several (three to four) times before transitioning to the next pose. Remember that remaining mindful and present with the sensations of movement and the breath is at the heart of practice. In our classes we often prepare the body for sitting meditation with yoga, but it's also fine to do sitting meditation first or let a yoga session stand on its own.

The entire sequence of lying or standing poses should take you at least twenty minutes to complete, but it could take much longer if you hold some postures for several breaths; if you zip through the postures much more quickly than that, you probably aren't moving mindfully with your breathing patterns. If you notice yourself doing this, take a moment to settle into the breath, and slowly continue.

Our group of teachers has also produced a CD with verbal instructions for these two series of movements. You can order them from the website: www.mindfulnesscalgary.ca.

PRACTICE 5.1
Lying Yoga Poses

1. *Rest pose:* Begin in rest pose. (See figure 5.1.)

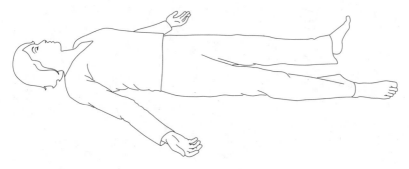

Figure 5.1 Rest Pose

2. Stretch your arms overhead and push your flexed feet away from the body, lengthening and stretching the entire body. (See figure 5.2.)

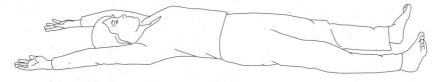

Figure 5.2 Lying Stretch

3. *Pelvic rocks:* On an outbreath, press your lower back into the floor, and rock on your tailbone, tucking your pelvis in toward your belly. (See figure 5.3.)

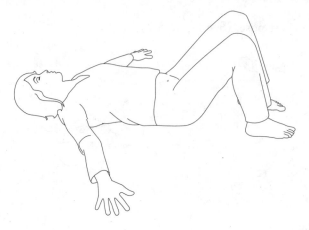

Figure 5.3 Pelvic Tilt Out

4. On an inbreath, rock your tailbone toward your feet, lifting your lower back and belly off the floor. (See figure 5.4.)

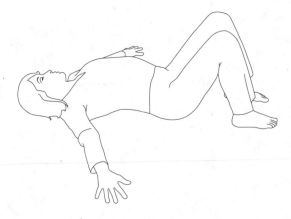

Figure 5.4 Pelvic Tilt In

5. *Thigh-to-chest stretch:* Pull your knees in toward your chest with both hands. Roll your knees around slightly to release your back muscles. (See figure 5.5.)

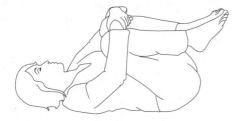

Figure 5.5 Knees to Chest

6. To intensify the stretch, lift your head as you exhale. Breathe in and slowly lower your head back to the floor. (See figure 5.6.)

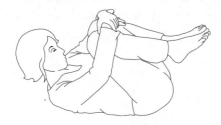

Figure 5.6 Head to Knees

7. *Hip-flexor stretch:* Lift your right knee toward your chest and hold with both hands, keeping your left leg stretched out on the floor. Then switch, stretching out your right leg and slowly lifting your left knee toward your chest. (See figure 5.7.)

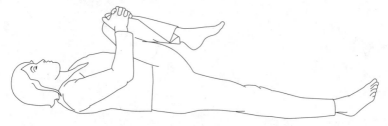

Figure 5.7 Knee to Chest with Extended Leg

8. To intensify the stretch on each side, lift your head toward your knee as you exhale. Breathe in as you slowly lower your head. (See figure 5.8.)

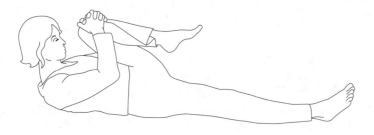

Figure 5.8 Head to Knee with Extended Leg

9. *Cat-cow stretch:* Begin in a neutral tabletop position on all fours with your back flat. (See figure 5.9.)

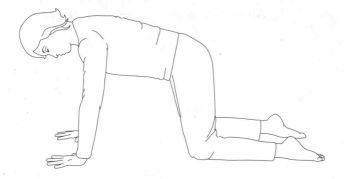

Figure 5.9 Hands and Knees

10. Breathe out, arching your back upward and dropping your head like a cat. (See figure 5.10.)

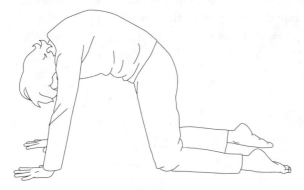

Figure 5.10 Cat Stretch

11. On an inbreath, allow your spine and belly to relax downward, and lift your head up like a swaybacked cow. Feel the movement begin at your tailbone and move up your spine in a wave to your neck and head. (See figure 5.11.) Alternately move between cat and cow.

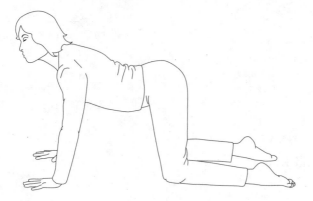

Figure 5.11 Cow Stretch

12. *Balancing pose:* Inhale and lift your right arm and left leg. Breathe deeply with the movement so that the breath supports the lift. Exhale and lower your arm and leg back to neutral position. Inhale and switch, lifting your left arm and right leg. (See figure 5.12.)

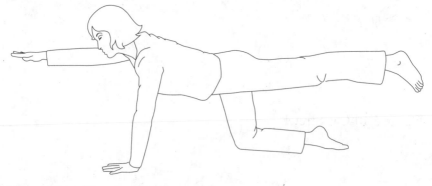

Figure 5.12 Hands and Knees Balancing

13. *Little bridge:* Mindfully return to rest pose, on your back. With an inbreath, raise your hands overhead, resting the backs of your hands on the mat. Then, lift your pelvis off the floor, using your thigh, back, and abdominal muscles. You could also do this with your hands by your sides. (See figure 5.13.)

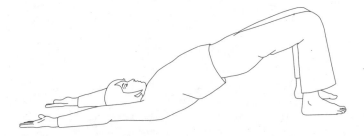

Figure 5.13 Little Bridge

14. *Spinal twist:* Place your hands, fingertips touching, behind your neck or extend your arms into a "T" position. As you exhale, drop your knees to one side and turn your head to the opposite side. Inhale as you raise your legs to the center, and exhale as you drop them to the other side and turn your head away. (See figure 5.14.)

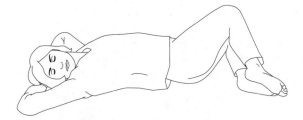

Figure 5.14 Lying Spinal Twist

15. *Leg lift:* Inhale and raise your left leg straight into the air, with your right knee bent and your right foot bracing the floor. Rotate your raised foot at the ankle. (See figure 5.15.)

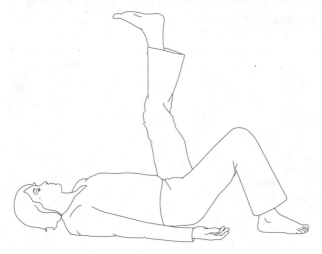

Figure 5.15 Leg Lift

16. Grab the back of your left calf or thigh, and gently ease your leg toward your head. (See figure 5.16.)

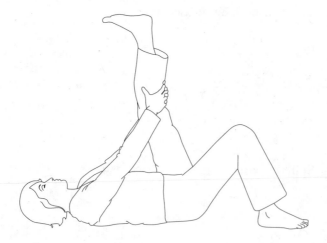

Figure 5.16 Leg Lift and Grab

17. If your body allows, as you exhale, lift your head toward your knee. Inhale as you slowly lower your head back to the floor. (See figure 5.17.) Repeat on the other side.

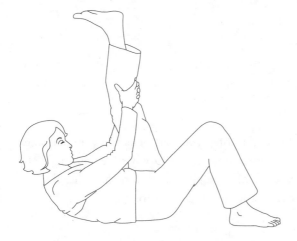

Figure 5.17 Leg Lift with Head Raise

18. *Side leg lift:* Lie on one side, supporting your head with your arm. Lift your top leg into the air as you inhale, with your toes pointing forward. Lower your leg slowly on the exhalation. Gently roll over and repeat on the other side. (See figure 5.18.)

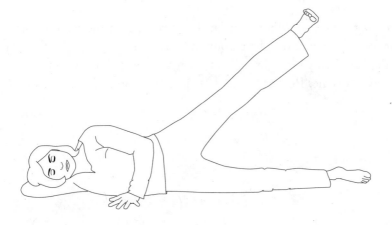

Figure 5.18 Side Leg Lift

19. *Lower cobra:* Lie on your front, with your arms down by your sides, and rest on your cheek or chin. (See figure 5.19.)

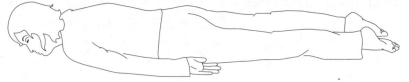

Figure 5.19 Lower Cobra Start

20. Bring your feet together and tighten your buttocks and your abdomen muscles. On an inbreath, look upward and slowly raise your head and upper trunk off the floor. Hold the pose for several breaths. Breathe out as you slowly lower to the floor. (See figure 5.20.)

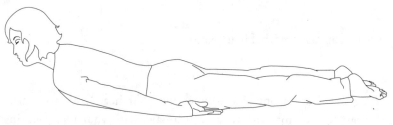

Figure 5.20 Lower Cobra Raise

21. *Beginning locust pose:* With your head still resting on the floor, bring your feet together and tighten your abdomen and buttocks. With an inhale, lengthen your right leg and lift it from your hip. Lower your leg as you exhale. Repeat on the left side. (See figure 5.21.)

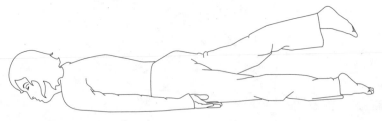

Figure 5.21 Beginning Locust

22. *Full locust pose:* For an added challenge, as you inhale, lift your head, trunk, and both legs off the floor all at the same time. (See figure 5.22.)

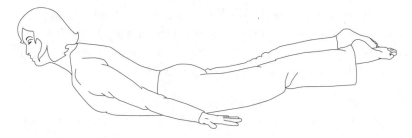

Figure 5.22 Full Locust

23. End the lying postures by returning to rest pose for five to ten minutes. Center your awareness on your breathing, observing the rise of your belly with each inbreath. Move your awareness through your body, sending the breath to any tight or sore areas. (Review figure 5.1.)

PRACTICE 5.2
Standing Yoga Poses

1. *Standing mountain pose:* Begin this sequence in standing mountain pose, with your arms by your sides, shoulders relaxed away from your ears, and feet parallel and about hip-width apart. Lengthen your body up through your spine. (See figure 5.23.)

2. Breathe in as you sweep extended arms out to the side and up toward the ceiling. Exhale as you lower them back down. (See figure 5.24.)

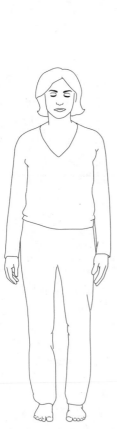

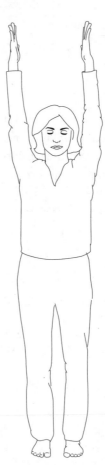

Figure 5.23 Standing
Mountain Pose

Figure 5.24 Standing with
Raised Arms

3. Inhale and raise your arms out to your sides. Pull your fingers up toward the ceiling and push out to the sides with your palms. Exhale and lower your arms back to your sides. (See figure 5.25.)

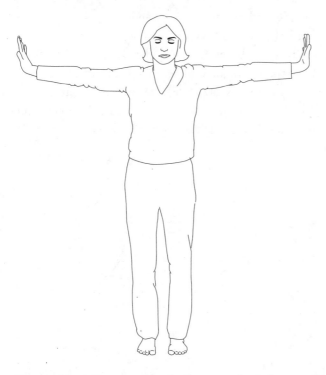

Figure 5.25 Standing with Outstretched Arms

4. Inhale and sweep one extended arm out to the side then up toward the ceiling while reaching down to the ground with the other arm. Exhale as you lower your arm. Repeat on the other side. (See figure 5.26.)

5. *Half-moon pose:* Inhale and sweep both extended arms out to the side then up toward the ceiling. As you exhale, bend to the side, as if you were sandwiched between two panes of glass. Maintain length through your spine. Inhale and reach up toward the ceiling again. Exhale and bend to the opposite side, with your arms still stretched overhead. With another inhale, return to the center, and as you exhale, lower your hands back to your sides. (See figure 5.27.)

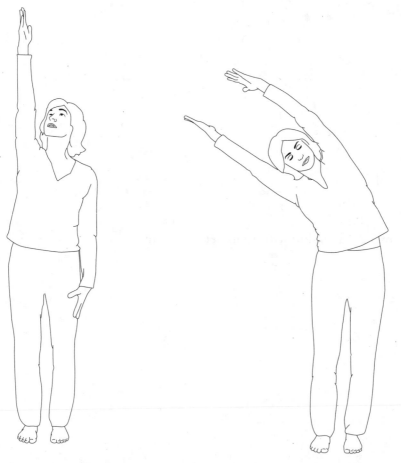

Figure 5.26 Standing
One-Arm Stretch

Figure 5.27 Half-Moon Pose

6. *Shoulder rolls:* Begin rolling your shoulders up and back, inhaling as you raise them up toward your ears, and then squeeze your shoulder blades together in back. Exhale as you let your shoulders drop, and squeeze your shoulders together in the front. Switch direction. (See figures 5.28 through 5.31.)

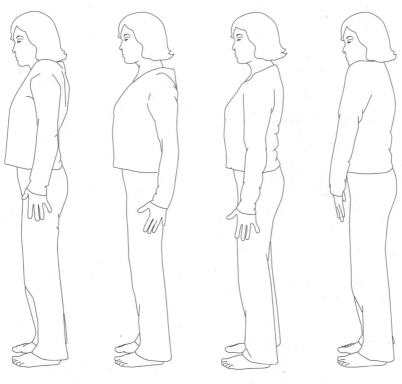

Figure 5.28
Shoulder Roll:
Up

Figure 5.29
Shoulder Roll:
Back

Figure 5.30
Shoulder Roll:
Down

Figure 5.31
Shoulder Roll:
Forward

7. *Neck rolls:* Allow your chin to fall toward your chest as you exhale, and then tilt your head to the right side so that your ear moves toward your shoulder. Inhale as you lengthen your neck, then tilt your head straight back, and finally tilt your head to the left so that your ear moves toward your shoulder. Rotate smoothly in one direction and then the other. (See figures 5.32 through 5.35.)

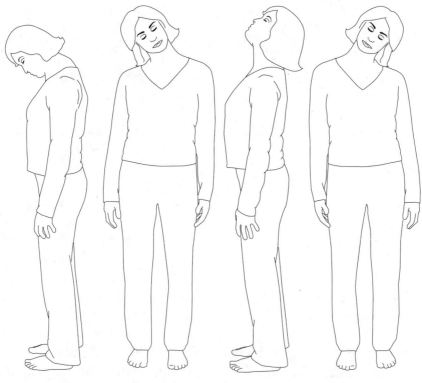

Figure 5.32
Neck Roll:
Forward

Figure 5.33
Neck Roll:
Right

Figure 5.34
Neck Roll:
Back

Figure 5.35
Neck Roll: Left

8. *Star pose:* Shift your weight onto one foot, and then, as you inhale, raise your arms to the sides and lift your other foot off the ground. Maintain the pose for several breaths and exhale as you return to standing. (See figure 5.36.)

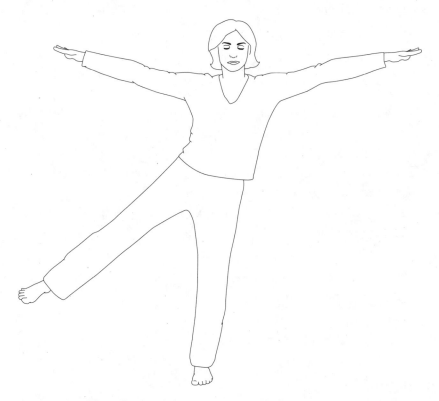

Figure 5.36 Star Pose

9. *Twist:* Lengthen your spine upward and inhale. Then, as you exhale, turn your body at the waist, rotate from the base of the spine, allow the twist to move up the spine, and complete the twist by turning your head to gaze over your shoulder. Repeat on each side. (See figures 5.37 and 5.38.)

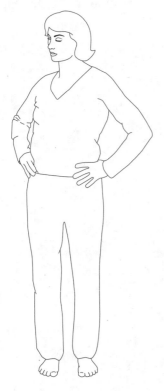

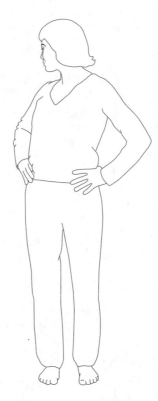

Figure 5.37 Standing Twist A   Figure 5.38 Standing Twist B

10. *Standing forward bend:* Bend your knees to enter and exit this pose. As you exhale, bend forward from the hips and allow your arms to dangle toward the floor. Place your hands on your thighs for support if needed. (See figures 5.39 and 5.40.)

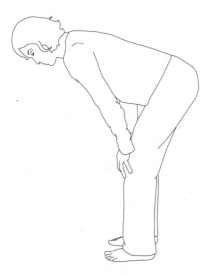

Figure 5.39 Standing
Forward Bend A

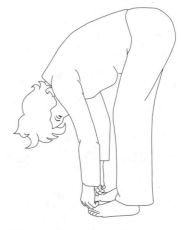

Figure 5.40 Standing
Forward Bend B

11. From the forward bending pose, come into a flat back posture as you inhale, reaching one arm in front, with the other on your thigh. Exhale back into the forward bend. Repeat on both sides. (See figure 5.41.)

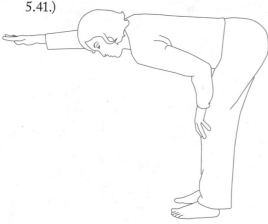

Figure 5.41 Standing Forward Bend with Extended Arm

12. *Chair pose:* From standing mountain pose, inhale, raising your arms in front of your body. With an exhale, bend at your knees as if you were sitting back into a chair, keeping your back straight and head upright. Hold for several breaths, if possible. Inhale as you stand back up, and exhale, dropping your arms back by your sides. (See figure 5.42.)

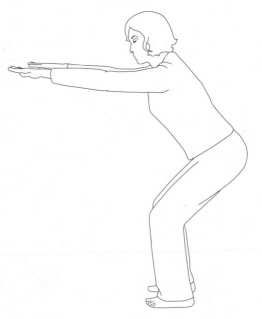

Figure 5.42 Chair Pose

13. *Tree pose:* Begin with your hands in prayer position in front of your body. Shift your weight onto one foot and place the sole of the other foot on your ankle, inside your calf, or on your upper thigh. When you are stable, reach your arms up. Repeat on both sides. (See figure 5.43.)

14. *Butterfly pose:* From a seated position, keep your back upright and bring the soles of your feet together. Relax your knees and thighs into the pose, without forcing them. Keep your shoulders relaxed and down. (See figure 5.44.)

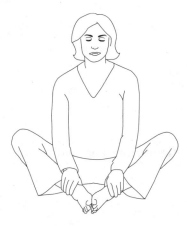

Figure 5.44 Butterfly Pose

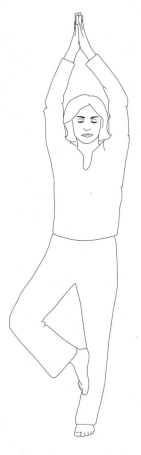

Figure 5.43 Tree Pose

15. *Forward bend:* With one leg outstretched and the other bent, sweep both arms out to the side and up toward the ceiling with an inhale, and fold forward from your waist as you exhale. Try not to hunch forward. Hold for several breaths. (See figures 5.45 through 5.47.)

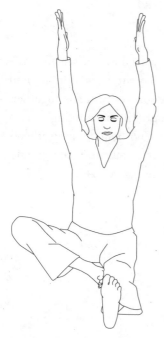

Figure 5.45 Forward Bend A

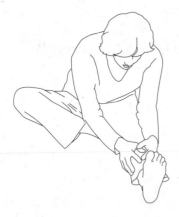

Figure 5.46 Forward Bend B

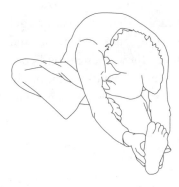

Figure 5.47 Forward Bend C

16. *Rest pose:* Finish your practice by returning to rest pose for five to ten minutes. (Review figure 5.1.)

WHEN TO PRACTICE YOGA

We often recommend doing some yoga before doing sitting meditation or body scan meditations to allow your body to become suppler, more alert, and relaxed before settling down into the stillness of meditation practice. Yoga can be great for getting going first thing in the morning, or even before bed to release some tension. Remember to always take into account your special needs or any sensitivity that may arise from bodily changes caused by cancer treatments like surgery, chemo, or radiation. If you have a sore arm from breast surgery, use caution in postures that require overhead stretching. Such stretches will assist your recovery, but be sure to proceed gently and follow your doctor's instructions.

If you practice these simple movements on a regular basis over the course of several weeks, you will begin to notice that the postures get easier and easier, you may move farther into the bends and twists, and you may discover that you have better balance. These changes will contribute to your recovery and help restore a sense of vitality. Above all, make sure your practice highlights awareness and never becomes just another exercise program.

CHAPTER 6

Balancing Breath

My life is not this steeply sloping hour,
In which you see me hurrying.
Much stands behind me; I stand before it like a tree;
I am only one of my many mouths,
And at that, the one that will be still the soonest.

I am the rest between two notes,
Which are somehow always in discord
Because death's note wants to climb over—
But in the dark interval, reconciled,
They stay there trembling.

And the song goes on, beautiful.

—Rainer Maria Rilke

In chapter 3 we talked about the importance of learning how to breathe deeply, using the diaphragm to fully inflate and deflate the lungs, which results in a full exchange of waste gases for oxygen and triggers the relaxation response. This chapter explains in more detail how this process works physiologically, then outlines several ways you can mindfully use the breath to help regulate your arousal levels on an everyday basis. The breath is an incredibly powerful tool that is always at your disposal and can be used to help you when you feel tired, stressed, or anxious.

Deep breathing can come in handy anytime you are facing stressful situations on your cancer journey, such as waiting for appointments, undergoing blood tests or scans, and even going through radiation or chemotherapy treatments. By learning a few basic principles about how the breath works and how you can mindfully modulate it, you will significantly add to your tool kit of coping techniques. People in our class have told us time and again that the breathing methods we teach are one of the things they use the most often, both during the program as they learn and practice meditation, and afterward, well into the future.

THE AUTONOMIC NERVOUS SYSTEM

The nervous system generally consists of two parts; one is under voluntary control, and the other is more automatic, called the *autonomic nervous system*. The voluntary part of the nervous system consists of the nerves that are used to produce intentional movement; for example, if you want to have a sip of your tea, you tell your arm to reach out and grab the handle of your cup. Then you tell your arm to bring it to your lips, and so on. All of this happens on a voluntary basis: you decide to make the movement, and your body responds. It may happen so quickly and seemingly without thought that it feels automatic, but it would not happen if you didn't will it first. Over the years, your body has learned to make these movements in response to your thoughts.

So the voluntary part of the nervous system refers to all those things that happen in response to your commands. But there are many things occurring in your body all the time that you don't specifically will; for example, your heart beats whether you tell it to or not, your lungs breathe, your glands secrete hormones, and your digestive system digests your food. It's a good thing, really! Can you imagine having to remember to do all of those things at every moment? So these "automatic" things are under the control of the autonomic nervous system, shown in figure 6.1; they happen whether we think about them or not.

The autonomic nervous system (the big "A" in the drawing) further consists of two parts, or arms: The *sympathetic nervous system* (*SNS*), which controls the stress response, and the *parasympathetic nervous system*

(*PNS*), which triggers the relaxation response. The SNS is the invigorating part of the system: when you feel that fight-or-flight reaction, that's the SNS kicking into high gear. The opposite of this is PNS activation: the relaxation response or rest phase. Your heart rate and breathing slow down, your muscles relax, and you feel calm. Your body may resemble that of a possum lying limp and relaxed. You can compare the SNS and PNS to the ends of a seesaw in that they balance each other out. When one arm is activated, the other is suppressed, and vice versa.

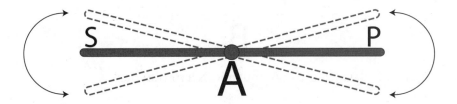

Autonomic Nervous System

Sympathetic	**Parasympathetic**
• fight or flight	• rest phase
• arousal	• possum
• activity	• relaxation

Figure 6.1 The Autonomic Nervous System

Balancing the Autonomic Nervous System

Despite being automatic, some aspects of the autonomic nervous system are also subject to voluntary control. Important in this context is the fact that you can control your breathing; you can purposely breathe more quickly or slowly, more shallowly or deeply. This turns out to be a really amazing and helpful thing! Simply put, each inbreath and outbreath corresponds with one arm of the autonomic nervous system, as shown in figure 6.2. Which goes with which?

Before you look for the solution, think about how you breathe when you are in a tense situation, scared or getting ready to face a physical challenge; do you sharply draw in a few deep breaths? Do you hold your breath? Do you start to hyperventilate (breathe faster)? These styles of breathing emphasize the inbreath, and ultimately stimulate the SNS, increasing arousal. Think about when the threat passes; you may heave a great sigh of relief or release. This type of breath emphasizes the outbreath. After practicing it a bit, you may be able to feel how the inbreath is the more arousing part of the breath, and the outbreath is the relaxing part.

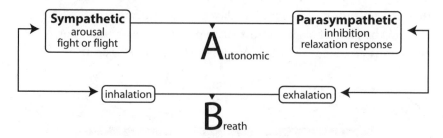

Figure 6.2 Balancing the Autonomic Nervous System

So if you take this knowledge of the inbreath as the invigorating part of the breath and the outbreath as the relaxing part, you can begin to consider how you could change the breath to suit your needs at any given time. For example, if you are lethargic and tired, but need to work or drive somewhere, you can use breathing that emphasizes the inbreath to increase your energy level. Conversely, if you feel stressed or anxious, you can use relaxing breaths that emphasize the outbreath to calm down.

Now we will show you a number of breathing practices that initially help you to balance out your stress and relaxation responses, and then focus more on either the relaxing or invigorating part of the breath. We call all of these practices "minis," for mini–breathing practices. This doesn't mean they are less important or useful than longer meditations but, rather, that they take only a few moments of your time. You can practice them almost anywhere and anytime.

"MINI" PRACTICES

For all the minis, the first step is to consciously switch to diaphragmatic breathing; take a few breaths to begin lengthening both your inbreaths and outbreaths. You will likely notice yourself sitting up straighter to allow the breath to penetrate deep into the belly. You may place your hand over your abdomen to feel the movement if that helps the breath deepen. Once you have established a good, deep belly breath, you can switch to the specific mini practices. The first few mini practices emphasize balancing or evening out the inbreath and the outbreath. It may take a bit of practice to get the rate of breathing just right for you. Don't approach this mechanically, make it into a struggle, or breathe so fast you begin to hyperventilate. Bringing awareness and sensitivity to your learning will help to refine your skills and knowledge.

Countdown Breathing

This is a very simple mini. After you have established deep breathing with even inbreaths and outbreaths, simply count down from ten to zero, using one count for each inbreath and outbreath. You can also imagine stepping down a step with each breath and becoming calm, yet aware and focused. This is a take on the common practice of stopping and counting to ten when you feel angry or irritated. You can do this just once, or repeat it if you have time or still feel upset.

Riding the Wave of Breath

For this mini, simply visualize a waveform that rises up with each inbreath and falls rhythmically with each outbreath. As you breathe in, count slowly in your mind from one to four. At the peak of the breath, when your lungs are comfortably full, begin to exhale slowly and count down from four to one. (See figure 6.3.) Try to make the breath flow smoothly and evenly, without any holding, gaps, or jerkiness.

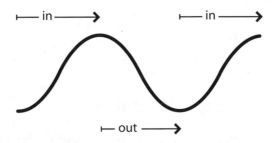

Figure 6.3 Wave Breath

Square Breathing

This mini also uses visualization, but in this case the breath takes the form of a square or possibly a rectangle. Instead of breathing in a smoothly flowing way, up and down like a wave, this time you hold the breath with mostly full or empty lungs, after both the inbreath and the outbreath. It may feel uncomfortable at first, but one tip is to make sure the lungs aren't totally empty or totally full when you pause; about 80 to 90 percent is good. Then, if it feels too difficult to hold for the same amount of time you breathed in or out, you can cut the time in half.

For example, in figure 6.4 the length of the pause is the same as the length of the breath, but you can also make the pause about half the length of the breath. The key to square breathing is to notice how the breath feels in the periods of stillness, and compare the stillness at the top of the breath, when your lungs are mostly full, to how it feels to pause in stillness when your lungs are emptied. These different feelings lead us into the next two breaths, which emphasize either the arousing or relaxing part of the breath.

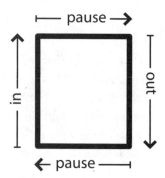

Figure 6.4 Square Breath

Relaxing Triangle Breathing

This practice takes into account the feeling of peacefulness and calm many people experience when they pause with mostly empty lungs after the exhalation. We call this a "triangular mini," because the breath follows a triangular pattern, which you can visualize as you breathe.

Simply inhale for a specified count (usually four), then immediately exhale for four counts, and finally hold for another two to four counts, or longer if it feels comfortable. This breath emphasizes the exhalation and therefore stimulates the relaxation response. Most people find this practice to evoke stillness and quiet once they get the hang of it.

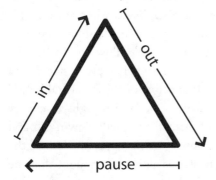

Figure 6.5 Triangle Breath

Invigorating Triangle Breathing

The opposite of the relaxing mini is the arousing mini, which takes the form of an upside-down triangle. Here, you pause only after the inhalation, which allows energy to build in your body as you hold the breath with mostly full lungs. If you are tired or feel low energy levels when you need to be active, this type of breathing practice can help.

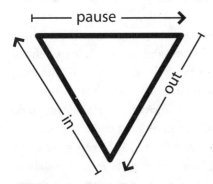

Figure 6.6 Inverted Triangle Breath

Alternate-Nostril Breathing

Originating from ancient yoga teaching and philosophy, the last breathing practice is based on a fundamental observation about the way people breathe. Can you tell right now whether you are breathing more through your left or right nostril? Do you think this is a ridiculous question? Most people look at us as if we have six heads when we ask this question, but the truth is that for the majority of people (unless you have some blockage or structural deformity that doesn't allow you to breathe through both nostrils), the dominant nostril switches every one and a half to two hours throughout the day. This is one of those natural bodily rhythms, similar to how most people have peaks and troughs in energy levels. The nervous system is organized such that signals flowing to and from one side of the body connect mainly to the opposite side of the brain. Because of this, when the left nostril is active it's thought that the right brain is more dominant. The right brain (at least, in most right-handed people) is known for being more receptive, creative, and relaxed than the left brain. Conversely, when the right nostril is dominant, this signals left-brain primacy, which means you are in a better state for active, intellectual pursuits. In left-handers, often the brain is wired in the opposite or a mixed pattern. In the yoga tradition, alternate-nostril breathing is said to balance sun and moon energies within us.

Regardless, have you figured out which of your nostrils is dominant right now? If you can't tell just by breathing, try blocking off one nostril and then the other to see which is easier to breathe through. Once you have figured this out, we will show you a practice that's great for balancing the autonomic nervous system and helping you feel clearheaded and energized.

Called *nadi shodhanam* in the yogic texts, alternate-nostril breathing is one of several ways of regulating the breath and energy that are refined in the yogic discipline known as *pranayama*. To set up for this practice, you need a way to comfortably rest your hand on your face so that you can manually close each of your nostrils. The most comfortable way to do this (although people often feel a bit silly at first—just make sure to do it for the first time in the privacy of your own home!) is to rest your index finger and middle finger of your right hand on your forehead just above your nose so that you can close off your right nostril with your thumb and your left nostril using your ring finger and little finger. Then follow the pattern of breathing shown in figure 6.7. Sit up straight so you can breathe deeply and fully. It might also help to blow your nose or rinse out your nasal passages before you begin.

In the first step, breathe in through both nostrils, then close the passive nostril (remember, you just figured this out), and exhale fully through just the active nostril. Then switch and close the active nostril, and inhale through just the passive nostril, and so on. After three full breaths of switching, you then both inhale and exhale through the passive nostril and switch sides for another three full breaths. This is one round, and we suggest you try three rounds to begin. Then lower your hand and breathe normally through both nostrils for a few breaths. What do you notice?

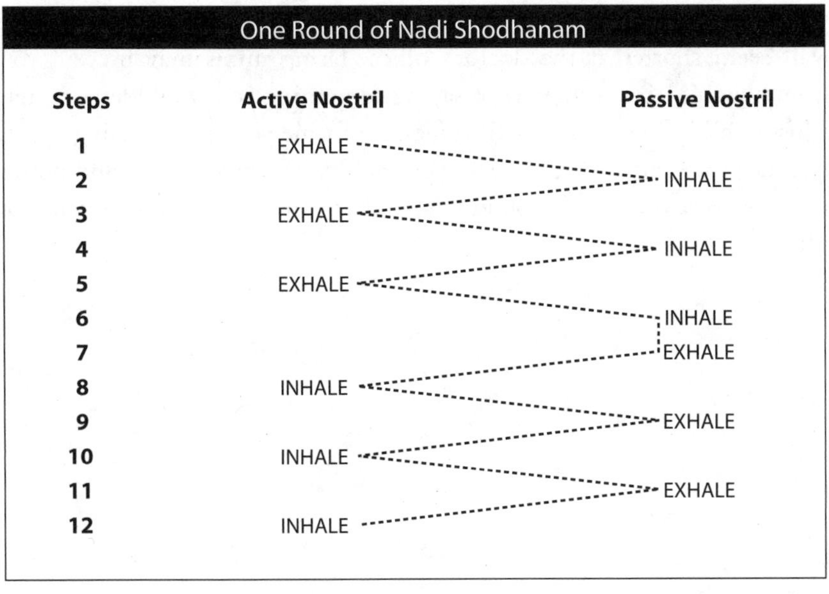

One Round of Nadi Shodhanam		
Steps	**Active Nostril**	**Passive Nostril**
1	EXHALE	
2		INHALE
3	EXHALE	
4		INHALE
5	EXHALE	
6		INHALE
7		EXHALE
8	INHALE	
9		EXHALE
10	INHALE	
11		EXHALE
12	INHALE	

Figure 6.7 Alternate-Nostril Breath

Most people find that once they get comfortable with the mechanics of this type of breathing, it tends to help clear the head. People describe feeling sharpness and clarity of mind, as well as often feeling energized. It's a good preparation for sitting meditation.

WHEN TO DO MINIS

There are no bad times to do minis. They result in your feeling more relaxed and in control of the situation, more patient and unhurried. You can do them with your eyes open or closed. Some preferred moments include sitting in traffic (red lights are particularly conducive to doing minis); waiting in shopping lines, waiting on hold on the phone, waiting for a phone call, or waiting in the doctor's office (you see the theme here); undergoing blood draws and medical tests; feeling bothered by something someone says; sitting in the dentist's chair; feeling overwhelmed by what you need to accomplish in the near future; being unable to sleep; feeling impatient and tempted to interrupt someone; and feeling pain. Pretty much anytime you think about doing a mini is a good time to do one.

There are many potential benefits: Minis may help to control the pain you experience during medical procedures, or they may help to make the wait seem shorter at the doctor's office. Using minis may prevent you from blowing up at someone or saying something you would later regret. Most of all, minis diminish the amount of time you spend feeling upset, frustrated, or impatient; increase your ability to pay attention and notice the beauty of the world around you; and enhance your overall quality of life.

CHAPTER 7

Stories We Tell Ourselves

In general, our understanding of any life event, including being diagnosed with cancer, is the outcome of mental processes wherein we create meaning from our raw experience. To make sense of unfolding events, we digest and integrate new events with our prevailing mental models or ideas of reality. In essence these models are like maps of experience that we have formed over a lifetime of learning and that we use to bring a sense of order and coherence to our lives. In this way, we continually revise our worldview as well as our understanding of where and how we, as individuals, fit into the bigger picture.

To clarify how all of this relates to stress and illness, as well as to your own capacity to enjoy happiness, peace, and tranquility in your life, it will help to take a closer look at this meaning-making activity and how your thoughts, beliefs, and expectations help to shape it.

YOUR LIFE IN STORIES

A special type of representation of reality you carry around with you is your personal narrative or life story. If someone asked you to talk about yourself, you would likely tell a story with a beginning, middle, and end. You'd probably say something about your family and where you were born or where you grew up. You might highlight certain key events in your life. You might talk about personal qualities you believe you possess, the kind of work you have done, and your personal interests or achievements. Who would any of us be without our stories?

In fact, this story-making proclivity is so pervasive that we could safely say it's a universal characteristic of human beings. We have or create stories to explain everything from large events like the creation of the universe or how the economy works to why we do what we do in any given situation.

One of the pitfalls of this storytelling, however, is that you actually might believe your stories. In fact most people usually do. We believe and act as if our stories are accurate depictions of reality, when in fact they never are. At best they are approximations or partial views of a reality that's so multifaceted, complex, and wonderful that it tends to defy description. Nevertheless we try to make sense of our experience, and the models, stories, beliefs, and such that we construct provide a rough map by which we live our lives. The thinking and imagining that underlie all this activity are undoubtedly very practical and necessary for living our lives day to day; however, there are a number of ways in which this story-making activity can lead us into trouble.

THE NATURE OF THOUGHT

The relative and subjective quality of thought as it relates to what's actually true or real has likely been recognized as long as human beings have walked the earth. It may have begun the first time a jungle vine was mistaken for a snake. One of the more familiar expressions of this issue is the famous line from Shakespeare's *Hamlet* (act 2, scene 2). In his response to Rosencrantz's objection to his likening of Denmark to a prison, Hamlet remarks, "Why, then, 'tis none to you; for there is nothing either good or bad, but thinking makes it so: to me it is a prison."

Commonly, we speak of a person who sees the glass as half full rather than half empty as an optimist, whereas the pessimist sees what's missing. Folk wisdom reminds us that every dark cloud has a silver lining. This commonplace understanding that our viewpoint can profoundly affect our experience has, in recent times, been subject to much scientific interest and scrutiny. As a result, it has become increasingly clear and certain that the interplay among thoughts, emotions, and behavior can have a powerful impact on your emotional health and overall well-being. Though simplistic notions about positive thinking have no place when you are facing cancer, it's useful to understand how your thinking may support or undermine your peace of mind and capacity to navigate the emotional minefield cancer may represent.

TROUBLE IN MIND: OUR DISTRESSING STORIES

Consider the following scenario: Margaret and Elise, two patients recently diagnosed with breast cancer, have met with their oncologists and received similar recommendations to proceed with a course of treatment that generally has very good outcomes. Objectively, from a medical standpoint, their situations are more or less the same.

Elise's thought process goes something like this: *Well, I don't expect this treatment to be easy, but I've been through tough times before, and I'm thankful that an effective treatment for this disease is available to me. My doctor was very supportive, and in balance, my chances look very good.* Meanwhile, Margaret's thought process goes somewhat differently: *I've heard horrible things about this treatment. Chances are I'm going to suffer quite a bit, and my doctor couldn't even guarantee that it will work. Things look pretty bleak, and this could be the end of me.*

You can see that the emotional consequences of these contrasting ways of viewing the same situation can be radically different. Though these scenarios are simplified for the sake of illustration, they very closely reflect actual disclosures shared repeatedly by patients like Margaret and Elise in our support groups. Not infrequently, both pessimistic and hopeful outlooks hold sway at different times within the same individual as the person struggles to make sense of what can be a confusing and possibly life-threatening predicament. And as normal and common as this emotional roller-coaster ride is, we wish to emphasize a few key points:

- Perception and appraisal are central determinants of your reaction to any challenging life event.

- You need not be a passive recipient, held helplessly captive by your potentially troubling and discouraging thoughts.

- Mindfulness has a key role to play in ensuring that you avoid unnecessary emotional suffering caused by troubling thoughts.

THOUGHTS RUNNING WILD

Within the field of psychology, a number of therapeutic approaches focus on how patterns of thinking influence mood, increase vulnerability to anxiety and depression, and impair effective functioning in the world. These patterns of thought can be close to the surface and easily available, such as the self-talk you typically engage in as you go about your day: *Oh, look what time it is; I'd better get a move on if I'm going to make my appointment*, or *Darn it, I guess I have to cook supper again! Why can't somebody else pitch in for a change?* You can probably recognize this self-talk as a kind of ongoing narrative voice in your head, judging and evaluating things as they occur. Thought patterns can also represent more covert, organized, and entrenched mental structures, sometimes referred to as *schemas*.

Schemas are very much like templates through which incoming sensory data is filtered to make sense of things. Because we match the data to fit our internal representations, they can be very powerful determinants of our experience. If we say that someone "looks at the world through rose-colored glasses" we are, in effect, talking about a schema that predisposes that person to put a positive spin on life conditions and events. Paying close attention over time to your own typical self-talk can give you clues that point the way to recognizing your own idiosyncratic schemas. Sometimes, it's easier for someone else to point out your schemas than for you to see them yourself, because to the person who has them, schemas are so ingrained that they are out of awareness and rarely questioned. It's very much like the way travelers discover things about their own culture when they go to another part of the world and bump up against other ways of seeing and doing. Assumptions about how the world works and how people relate to each other may no longer apply.

One of the problems with using these automatic modes of processing experiences is that your body reacts to the stories the voice in your head tells, whether the stories are accurate or not. Thoughts that result in alarming ideas create alarm in your body through your stress reaction, and if you chronically engage with distorted and distressing thoughts, your body can become chronically harnessed to that type of thinking. Over time such thinking can lead to fear, chronic stress, self-blame, and depression. People can become so entrenched in the worry habit that they practically become worry machines.

Pitfalls in Thinking

Distorted cognitions, dysfunctional thinking, and maladaptive schemas are a few of the terms used in psychology to describe the human tendency to bias perceptions and judgments based on limitations of our prevailing inner representations of reality. We are prone to be misled by our thinking in a number of characteristic ways, summarized with some of the following examples.

Labeling or stereotyping: Seeing people or situations as fixed and unchanging, and ignoring other aspects or possibilities; for example, *My doctor is uncaring* or *Women are the weaker sex.*

Jumping to conclusions: Making an interpretation in the absence of clear evidence to support it; for example, when your doctor fails to mention a test result, you conclude, *The results must be bad*; or when a friend fails to return a phone call, you determine, *She doesn't want to talk to me; she must be mad at me.*

Magnification (catastrophizing) and minimization: Exaggerating the importance or likelihood of something seen as negative, or minimizing the importance or likelihood of something seen as positive; for example, *It's terrible and unbearable that my doctor recommends another treatment* or *My accomplishments don't amount to much.*

Emotional reasoning: Believing that it must be true because you feel it or fear it; for example, the oncologist spends only a few moments with you during a clinic visit, so you think, *I feel uncared for; my oncologist doesn't like me*; or when you notice your fear, you think, *If I have negative thoughts, my disease will return.*

Mental filters: Picking out a limited aspect of a situation or experience and allowing it to color your perception of the whole event; for example, you have a hard time finding parking at the hospital, so *The hospital is a horrible place.*

All-or-nothing thinking: Seeing everything in black-and-white categories; for example, your spouse doesn't help clean up after dinner, so you declare, "I do everything around here. You don't care about me at all!" or you receive an unwelcome test result, so you think, *Nothing ever goes right for me!*

Personalization: Interpreting an event as being about you when there are many other plausible causes or interpretations; for example, someone you know initially walks in your direction but, after getting closer, suddenly turns and walks the other way, so you think, *That person dislikes me and was trying to avoid me.*

Musterbation (perfectionism): Thinking that you "must" or "should" behave in a certain way or else!—often combined with an unrealistic conclusion regarding the consequences of failing to do it; for example, *I must be a good patient, or my doctor won't give me the attention I need* or *I must keep up appearances, or others will see my imperfections and reject me.*

Mindfulness for Observing Thoughts

Mindfulness allows you to more readily recognize when you are engaging in these thinking pitfalls so you can see the limitations they may impose on your life. This gives you the possibility of choice, whereas previously you may have reacted automatically. It can help to identify and challenge assumptions and distortions in your thinking so you can obtain a more balanced understanding of a situation. This may allow new solutions, possibilities, or feelings to emerge. When you become aware of engaging in these forms of thinking:

- Realize that thoughts are just thoughts; they are not reality. As scientist and philosopher Alfred Korzybski said, "The map is not the territory."

- Remember that you are not your thoughts; they arise and pass away like waves on the ocean. You are more like the ocean than the waves.

Here are some helpful questions you might ask yourself:

- *How do I know that my assumption is true; what's the evidence?*

- *Are there any other possible explanations or ways of seeing it?*

- *Even if it's true, are the consequences necessarily as horrible as I feel they are?*

- *Is this really the most helpful interpretation, or are there other possible explanations I could more readily accept that would allow other courses of action?*

- *Just because something may be true at one time or in one situation, does that mean it will always be true?*

- *Are there exceptions to the rule and new possibilities I might use to guide my behavior, rather than allow my self-limiting beliefs to guide it?*

Realize that whether or not thoughts are accurate, engaging in rumination steals you away from the beauty and possibility inherent in the present moment.

PRACTICE 7.1
Challenging Your Assumptions

Using the following chart as an example, take a blank sheet of paper and work through a difficult situation. You will know it's a good time to do this practice when you find yourself having a strong emotional reaction to a situation. Your reaction may seem excessive even to yourself. Working through this chart can help you understand your reaction and your options in the situation.

SITUATION Describe the events surrounding an unpleasant emotional experience. List just the facts, as a video camera might capture, without any interpretation.	EXAMPLE RESPONSES *Friend walked by me on the sidewalk without acknowledging me.*
EMOTIONS Describe the emotion aroused, such as anger, sadness, or fear, and how strong it is on a scale from 1 to 10.	*Hurt (10), rejection (8), anger (6)*
AUTOMATIC THOUGHTS What thoughts can you identify that preceded or contributed to the negative emotion?	*She ignored me on purpose.* *She knows I have cancer; she's avoiding me because of that.* *She probably doesn't want to have anything to do with me anymore.* *How dare she turn on me in my time of need?*
DISTORTIONS OF THOUGHT Identify the possible distortions or limitations in each automatic thought from the list of "Pitfalls in Thinking" in the previous section.	*Jumping to conclusions, magnification, personalization, catastrophizing.*
ALTERNATIVE RESPONSE How could you think or behave differently in the situation?	*Maybe she didn't see me.* *Maybe she had something else on her mind.* *Maybe she's avoiding me because she doesn't know what to say.* *I could call her and find out what's going on.*

OUTCOME	
How would you feel or behave if you substituted the alternative response for the automatic thought? Has the emotional intensity shifted?	*Diminished feelings of hurt, rejection, and anger.* *Empowered myself by taking action to find out what was really happening.*

THE "DON'T KNOW" MIND

While the previous practice highlights how mindfulness can help you gain perspective on disquieting thoughts and enable you to work with them, perhaps a more profound insight comes when you recognize that thoughts are just thoughts. When you can gain that understanding through your practice, becoming an impartial witness to your own mental process, you weaken the stranglehold your thoughts may have on you. You can choose to identify less with what has sometimes been called "roof-brain chatter" (Pearce 1974), that incessant self-talk of the cerebral cortex, or "roof" of the brain. With practice you may find that you have less of a compulsive need to render judgments or come to inflexible conclusions. The mind that's uncluttered with thought—that is, marked by the spacious clarity and openness that emerges when thought subsides—is the beginner's mind discussed in chapter 3. It has also been called "quiet mind" or "don't know mind." In a sense, the mind that doesn't know, that doesn't succumb to the illusion of knowing that thoughts encourage, is a wise mind, a mind that can transcend stale and conventional views, a mind that's more attuned to the wonder of life as it unfolds and a mind that's at peace.

WALKING MEDITATION

When, around the midpoint of the program, we first introduce mindful walking to our classes, sometimes there's a bit of confusion. Many people have taken to walking for mild or moderate exercise or just as a way to get away from it all, to get out into nature and leave their worldly cares behind. Walking is also a favorite venue for daydreaming, problem solving, or chatting with friends. Though these types of experiences can be rewarding and enjoyable, mindful walking is something altogether different. Mindful walking meditation is a way to begin to move mindfulness off the meditation cushion and out into the world. In this way it can act as a bridge to bringing greater presence to all of your activities and experiences.

You can do it anywhere there's enough room to stand and take a few steps in a given direction. Traditionally, walking meditation is often done in a prescribed space, such as in a lane, back and forth. Unlike your usual walking, there is no destination, except to be fully present in the here and now of each step. Simply follow the instructions in practice 7.2, next.

PRACTICE 7.2
Mindful Walking Meditation

Begin by standing comfortably erect and in balance. Clarify your intention before you start walking: to walk and be completely present and aware of what the senses convey of the experience in each moment and in each step as you take it.

Initially, in relative stillness—simply sensing the body standing in balance and breathing—following the custom of clasping the hands in front of or behind the body—slowly and deliberately, the arms not swinging in counterpoise to the walking gait as when walking to get somewhere—gazing out in front a number of paces with soft focus, to see without looking—not needing to gaze down at the feet—instead sensing where they are—realizing that they know how to walk.

When clarity and focus are present—beginning to take the first step and sensing what's happening—noticing how the weight initially shifts onto one foot, lifting the other foot, moving the leg and foot forward, and placing the foot down on the ground—now, beginning the next step with a shift of weight to the newly planted foot—attending to each step with openness, curiosity, and wonder.

Perhaps noticing a soft smile of appreciation and gratitude for this opportunity to practice finding expression on the face—noting inwardly

118

each phase of the step—shifting, lifting, reaching, placing—helping sustain mindfulness throughout.

On reaching the end of the prescribed space—stopping—being aware of stopping—beginning to turn—being aware of turning—and beginning anew.

These being the basic instructions in their simplest form, knowing that many variations are possible—perhaps slowing the steps—shifting from the usual pace of walking—helping break the habit of walking without awareness—or walking faster—perhaps enjoying coordinating the rhythm of the steps with the flow of breath such that each inbreath and outbreath has a given number of steps associated with it—extending this awareness to include various aspects of the ongoing experience, just as for sitting meditation— of course, attention may wander, so noticing this, bringing it back again without judgment or derision—simply returning awareness—pausing— beginning anew with the next step—instead of noting lifting, reaching, or placing, possibly thinking other words, like here, now, alive, wonderful— *whatever helps keep awareness focused and alive.*

Knowing that another variation may be to take this walking out into the world—with the same clarity of intention present in each step—hearing sounds—seeing shifting shapes and colors, and feeling the wind on the face and contact with the earth in each step—again, whenever noticing that consciousness has drifted off into identifying, thinking, analyzing, or judging mode—dropping the thought where it was found, like an old, useless stick— beginning anew—remembering, no goal or destination is involved other than to be fully present—and each moment when you are fully present, you have arrived.

One man in our classes began practicing informal walking meditation on his way to work in the morning. He had previously made walking to work part of his healthy lifestyle, but typically became absorbed in thinking and worrying about anticipated difficulties at work that day. How did walking mindfully change things? He said he started to notice that there were certain people he predictably encountered each day on his walk, a fact of which he had been totally oblivious. He began to greet them, share a smile, and sometimes converse with them. He felt it created a more pleasant start to each day of his life in the workaday world.

Thinking can have such a hold on our minds that taking some time to intentionally step out of the trance of thought, through formal and informal meditation practices, can be liberating, over time helping us begin to recognize the distinction between thoughts and raw experience. In your day-to-day life, you can begin to notice and challenge unhelpful beliefs and assumptions. You can practice withholding or tempering your judgments as a path to seeing things more clearly and in a broader context.

HOW TO PRACTICE THESE SKILLS

Especially when you find yourself reacting strongly to a situation, try to become aware of the dance between your thoughts and feelings. Begin to recognize the possibility of responding skillfully rather than reacting out of unhelpful thought habits. With practice, you may find that you can free yourself from unhelpful thinking patterns you may have acquired.

At this point in your practice, we suggest beginning to alternate or mix in the walking meditation with daily sitting meditation and yoga stretches. You might, one day, do fifteen minutes of lying yoga followed by thirty minutes of walking meditation and, the next day, try fifteen minutes of standing yoga followed by thirty minutes of sitting meditation. As you progress through the program, we suggest trying to increase your time spent in formal practice to forty-five minutes each day.

CHAPTER 8

Meditation with Imagery

Wild Geese

You do not have to be good.

You do not have to walk on your knees

For a hundred miles through the desert, repenting.

You only have to let the soft animal of your body love what it loves.

Tell me about despair, yours, and I will tell you mine.

Meanwhile the world goes on.

Meanwhile the sun and the clear pebbles of the rain

Are moving across the landscapes,

Over the prairies and the deep trees,

The mountains and the rivers.

Meanwhile the wild geese, high in the clean, blue air,

Are heading home again.

Whoever you are, no matter how lonely,

The world offers itself to your imagination,

Calls to you like the wild geese, harsh and exciting—

Over and over announcing your place

In the family of things.

—Mary Oliver

Within our mindfulness-based approach, imagery is used as a way to encourage, strengthen, and remind us of beneficial qualities and capacities that are intrinsic to our nature, yet often underdeveloped or obscured by suffering, negative expectations, or perceptual habits.

Our approach differs quite a bit in emphasis from one that's frequently advised for cancer patients: that is, focusing on achieving specific goals or outcomes through visualization. Such an approach may have its place, but its goal-driven and outcome-oriented striving can be counterproductive to mindfulness practice. In our way of thinking about it, healing cannot be forced or willed, yet we can play a role in creating conditions that support its underlying processes.

In the broader context of cultivating nondoing and nonstriving, you can use imagery to heighten your awareness of aspects of being that are life affirming, beneficial, and even inspirational.

YOUR LIFE IN IMAGES

Take a moment to consider that imagery is a potent force in your life. Images are representations of the world that influence our experience in a way similar to language. When we use the word "imagery," we include representations in all of our sensory channels, not only the visual. In chapter 2 we suggested that you imagine biting into a lemon wedge to experience firsthand a bodily response to mental activity. For most people, imagining the act of sampling a lemon in all sensory channels—the lemon's citrus smell; the rind's waxy, nubbly texture; the brilliant-yellow color; and the taste of the glistening, juice-filled flesh—produces a very strong response in the digestive tract that may be most evident by a puckering mouth and gushing saliva.

What kind of response do you feel inside when you imagine the face of a dearly loved friend or family member? What about when you imagine a situation you would prefer to avoid, such as rushing to catch a plane or being confronted by an angry person? If you consider it carefully, you may recognize that you generate internal representations of the world fairly routinely as you move through your day and that even in sleep, images in the form of dreams can be powerfully evocative. Some images are so rooted in the human imagination that they are considered to be *archetypal*, commonly shared images that capture some fundamental aspect of human experience, such that they become universal symbols shared across cultures.

For example, people living near high mountains have often regarded them as sacred, and climbing a mountain is easily recognized as a metaphor for a spiritual quest. It's not surprising that mountains, where the beauties of earth and sky meet in stark conjunction, have the power to move people on many levels.

MOUNTAIN MEDITATION

Mountain meditation, introduced by Jon Kabat-Zinn in his excellent book *Wherever You Go, There You Are* (1994), offers a path to insight about aspects of your own nature that you would do well to recognize and honor. At some point you might enjoy practicing mountain meditation outdoors, where the elements provide reminders of our direct kinship with the natural world.

Practice 8.1 presents instructions for "Mountain Meditation," and you can approach using these instructions in various ways. You could have a friend read them to you, you could make a recording of them to play back, or you could simply read them and use your general sense of the instructions as a basis for inwardly guiding your own mountain meditation.

PRACTICE 8.1
Mountain Meditation

You can do mountain meditation in any position, yet a seated posture may be most apt because the seated body bears formal resemblance to a mountain: broad at the base and tapering to the sky.

Begin by taking your seat. Whether that's on the floor or a cushion, or in a chair, allow your body to settle into a comfortable, balanced, and stable position. You may rest your hands on your knees or fold them in your lap. A comfortably erect spine can bring a sense of dignified purpose to your meditation, encouraging an alert state of mind. At the same time, refrain from enforcing excessive rigidity, tension, or stiffness. Your eyes may be open or closed, but many people find it easier to prime the imagination with closed eyes, and you'll have less competition from visual stimuli around you.

Bringing awareness to sensing the body—taking a few moments to become aware of the symphony of sensations emanating from your being that announce the existence of the body—while tuning in to bodily sensations— allowing the opportunity to soften or release areas where unnecessary tension may have taken residence outside of awareness.

Calling to mind the image of a mountain—perhaps a familiar one—a mountain whose image has been captured in memory or a completely original, imagined creation that represents all a mountain can be—taking a moment to envision the mountain's overall form—single or many-peaked—and whether it's glacier-topped, covered in snow, or forested—appreciating the beauty, strength, and dignity the mountain embodies.

Once this image is established—letting the sense of becoming the mountain develop—mountain and body becoming one—legs and pelvis becoming mountain's sturdy base, firmly rooted in the earth's crust—spine becoming mountain's axis—torso and arms the sloping mountainside—head and shoulders the majestic peak—the mountain's enduring quality becoming that of the body.

While sitting in mountain stillness—allowing the surrounding world to shift and change—with sunrise, the dawn's soft light moving across the mountain's face, burning the dew off its lower slopes—shadows shifting and changing while the sun is moving higher in the sky, and mountain streams being refreshed by the day's new glacial melt—animals moving into the meadows to enjoy the forage and the sun's warmth—and in this manner, morning shifting into midday—day into moonlit night—and night into day—throughout the shifting cycles—mountain sitting unmoved—beautiful and stable in its equipoise.

Through the seasons, too, the mountain endures—while spring flowers are giving way to summer lushness and heat—the mountain is bearing witness—soon the greens of summer foliage are surrendering into the fall palette of brilliant yellows, reds, and oranges and muted shades of brown— weather is chilling toward fall—daylight hours are shortening—and perhaps rain, ice, and snow are pelting the mountain—perhaps birds and animals are migrating, moving from high meadows to protected valleys—perhaps those visiting the mountain are judging it based on the placid weather or the good views—yet the mountain remains unaffected by such judgments—mountain sits calmly in its majesty—abiding all change.

Now sitting in your own mountain nature—perhaps receiving from the mountain some of its gifts—perhaps recognizing the stable and enduring elements within your own being, even as all that surrounds is shifting and changing.

As the storms, shifting weather, and seasons of your own life move through their rhythms, may the timeless wisdom of the mountain remain close at hand.

LAKE AND TREE MEDITATIONS

The mountain is just one image from nature that can help during your meditation practice. A wide variety of natural images can help emphasize qualities you may want to strengthen in yourself. Another common practice, also introduced by Jon Kabat-Zinn in *Wherever You Go, There You Are* (1994), is to imagine the qualities of a lake: when still and calm, the lake's surface acts as a mirror, reflecting the light of the world around it. When you embody this quality of the lake, your calmness and stillness allow you to be a mirror that reflects with clarity and transparency. With this clarity, you can look both inward to your own depths and rich inner resources, and outward to see the world with a clarity unveiled by illusion.

Additionally, when the lake's surface becomes choppy or rough from wind and rain, you only have to descend gently to the lake's depths, where this turbulence is reduced to a rhythmic swaying current, akin to the flow of breath. Hence, even in the midst of stormy weather on the surface, the lake's depths remain quiet and calm and can be a place of refuge or comfort in your own life's storms. The tree image appeals to the same principle: though the tree's branches may whip about in a storm and its leaves may be torn off, its trunk only sways slightly and its roots reach deep into the earth to provide stability.

Each of these images can help you feel rooted and calm in the midst of the inevitable storms of life that can whip up at a moment's notice. Recognizing or imagining yourself as calm as the depths of the lake, strong and unmoving like the mountain, or rooted like the tree can help you more easily weather these storms.

USES OF NATURE MEDITATION

You can use these imagery-based meditations anytime you formally practice meditation or even during informal meditation times, whenever you feel vulnerable, small, or fragile.

Bill, a prostate-cancer patient who came to our classes, was enduring a "watchful waiting" period. When he had learned that no immediate treatment was recommended, he had begun to compulsively and frequently check his PSA (prostate specific antigen) levels, a rise in which might indicate that the cancer was growing. He shared that he felt as if he were just waiting for an increase that would signal his cancer's progression.

As if this wasn't nerve-racking enough, he also described often feeling overwhelmed by the demands of his job as a midlevel city bureaucrat; he frequently felt overlooked, taken for granted, or trampled on by his superiors. Using the image of the mountain helped Bill in both circumstances. As a cancer patient just waiting for things to get better or worse, he could embody the mountain's qualities of equanimity and endurance over incredibly long periods of geological time to practice patiently accepting the uncertainty of his situation. At work, he could raise himself up and feel majestic, solid, and unaffected, thinking of the mountain even in the face of insults or put-downs. The mountain's qualities of freedom, space, and majesty helped him rise above office politics and do his job with pride.

You, too, can likely find times in your life when reminding yourself of your mountainlike attributes helps you endure uncertainty, long waits, external evaluations, or assaults on your integrity. Embodying mountain qualities in these situations can help affirm your strength and endurance during these difficult times.

CHAPTER 9

A Day of Silence

Love After Love
The time will come
when, with elation,
you will greet yourself arriving
at your own door, in your own mirror,
and each will smile at the other's welcome,

and say, sit here. Eat.
You will love again the stranger who was your self.
Give wine. Give bread. Give back your heart
to itself, to the stranger who has loved you

all your life, whom you ignored
for another, who knows you by heart.
Take down the love letters from the bookshelf,

the photographs, the desperate notes,
peel your own image from the mirror.
Sit. Feast on your life.

—Derek Walcott

Between weeks six and seven of our eight-week MBCR program, we offer a unique opportunity for participants to take time out from their usual busy schedules to spend six hours in silence, simply nurturing themselves. Six hours isn't that much time, really, but it's amazing how difficult people find it to carve out that segment of their Saturday just for their own reflection and well-being. People are often intimidated initially by the idea of meditating for six hours straight. They may also wonder how they could go for that long surrounded by people without speaking. After they do it, though, the comments we hear the most are "The time just flew by," and "Because we did so many different forms of meditation and yoga, nothing seemed overwhelming." Participants often tell us the silence was refreshing and much easier to sustain than they thought it would be.

We really hope you will also take up this challenge and plan a quiet day of meditation for yourself! It doesn't have to follow the schedule or format we will describe; in fact it can be quite different, but the important thing is to set aside this larger chunk of time just to practice mindfulness, preferably in silence, either alone or with others who are also participating. You will be amazed at what you will find if you commit to giving this a try!

WHY PRACTICE A DAY OF MINDFULNESS IN SILENCE?

Given your multitude of choices for spending your valuable and increasingly precious time, why would you spend the better part of a day by yourself, meditating in silence? Choosing to set aside an extended period of time truly represents a commitment to yourself and the healing process, reinforcing the importance of mindful practice in your life. It offers a chance to become more intimate and familiar with the comings and goings of your own bodymind, continuing your process of befriending yourself. It represents time for quiet, individual reflection and slowing down the harried pace of everyday life. It simplifies life at an often busy and rushed time, and it also strengthens your ability to be mindful and concentrate for prolonged periods.

In shorter daily meditation sessions, you don't often get a chance to sustain your concentration for such a long period; there's no other way to learn this but by extending the length of practice. In addition, with increasing proficiency, it takes longer for learning opportunities to arise in meditation, but you can rest assured that over the span of the day, you will likely get an opportunity to work with many of the challenging emotions and thoughts you would probably like to address.

But Why Silence?

We choose to meditate in silence for a number of reasons. Language, a form of symbolic representation of experience, relates to thoughts, beliefs, and ideas, and it tends to remove us from present-centered awareness. It takes us one step farther away from the bare awareness we are trying to cultivate. Silence, in contrast, allows you to be closer to your bare awareness and also to focus concentration and conserve energy for the work of mindfulness. Talking and sociability with others requires considerable energy output that we would like you to direct toward your personal practice for this time span. In group practice, we apply what's known as "noble silence," which comes from traditional meditation practices and includes maintaining not only silence but also "custody of the eyes," so that if you are practicing with others, you refrain from making eye contact or communicating in other nonverbal ways. It may seem awkward at first, but if everyone is following this directive, you will find that it feels quite freeing after a time. This time in silence allows you to practice just being with things as they are, and accepting these things without the outlet or entanglement of communicating with others. Both the silence and length of time allow for deep personal exploration and development of insight.

WHAT THE DAY INVOLVES

Our silent retreat day weaves together practices learned over the course of the program, including yoga, body scan, sitting and walking meditation, eating meditation, and the use of poetry. We also usually incorporate some other practices, such as chanting or using sound meditation with singing bowls. Here's a sample schedule:

9:00–9:15	Welcome, introduction, and ground rules
9:15–9:45	Lying yoga
9:45–10:10	Body scan
10:10–10:20	Break
10:20–10:50	Sitting choiceless-awareness meditation
10:50–11:20	Standing or walking meditation
11:20–11:50	Mountain, lake, or tree meditation
11:50–12:00	Break
12:00–12:45	Eating meditation
12:45–1:15	Walking meditation
1:15–1:40	Sound meditation: lying, chanting, bowls
1:40–1:50	Break
1:50–2:20	Standing yoga or partnered yoga
2:20–2:45	Sitting loving-kindness meditation
2:45–3:00	Reflection with partners, final meditation, closing circle

There are a number of elements in this schedule that we have not yet introduced to you in the book, including eating meditation; although you did this with the raisin in chapter 3, now you will get a chance to do it with your entire lunch. The principle's the same: eat slowly with awareness of each bite. Before you even bite into your food, observe it with all your senses: sight (note the colors, shape, nuance of reflected light), smell, sound, and texture. Note the sound as you take each bite. Chew each mouthful thoroughly, noticing the variety of tastes as they make their way around your mouth. Wait until you have completely finished with each mouthful before lining up the next one. We usually allocate about forty-five minutes to this eating meditation, but you can certainly take longer if you like.

We also incorporate the mountain meditation you learned in the last chapter into the day of silence; sometimes we use a lake or tree meditation instead. These meditations share the approach of using an image from nature to help you embody the qualities of a natural object as you practice mindfulness meditation.

Loving-Kindness Meditation

Another form of meditation we introduce in the silent retreat is loving-kindness meditation. Traditionally called *metta meditation*, loving-kindness is one of several practices that aims to help you nurture a specific quality through meditation practice. The practice of loving-kindness meditation traditionally takes many months or years to fully develop. You begin slowly, by cultivating wishes for either your own or your closest loved ones' happiness. Then the circle very gradually expands to include wishes for the well-being of more-distant friends, acquaintances, and strangers; eventually even your enemies; and finally all living beings.

One of North America's foremost experts and teachers of metta practice, Sharon Salzberg, of the Insight Meditation Society in Barre, Massachusetts, has written several excellent books on this topic, including *Lovingkindness: The Revolutionary Art of Happiness* (1995) and *A Heart as Wide as the World: Stories on the Path of Lovingkindness* (1997), both from Shambhala Publications. We recommend consulting these books for more-detailed background and instructions on this type of practice. We have adapted the following instructions from *Insight Meditation: A Step-by-Step Course on How to Meditate*, an audio kit by Sharon Salzberg and Joseph Goldstein (2002).

PRACTICE 9.1
How to Practice Loving-Kindness Meditation

Sit comfortably and relax as much as possible. Don't try to force anything or make anything special happen, and don't try to contrive extraordinarily loving feelings. Just relax, be at ease, and sit comfortably. Imagine that you are out in a big, wide, open field, just planting seeds of intention.

1. Begin metta meditation by opening to yourself and directing a sense of loving care, friendship, kindness, and connection to yourself. Simply rest your mind in the awareness of your wish to be happy, which is rightful, appropriate, and beautiful. You, like all beings everywhere, simply want to be happy. Perhaps consider the many ways you have suffered through your experience with cancer, and consider your genuine wish to emerge from this experience feeling happy and whole.

    There are four traditional phrases for metta meditation: *May I be free from danger* or *May I live in safety*, *May I be happy*, *May I be healthy*, and *May I live with ease*.

    Living with ease refers to allowing day-to-day life activities, like family and work, to go easily: *May it not be a struggle*. Let each phrase emerge from your heart, and connect to it; simply connect to it, without trying to force any special feeling or make anything happen.

    May I be free from danger, *May I be happy*, *May I be healthy*, *May I live with ease*—you can develop a rhythm that's pleasing to you. You don't have to hurry. There can be space or silence. Once again, let the phrases emerge: *May I be free from danger*, *May I be happy*, *May I be healthy*, *May I live with ease*. Continue with these wishes for your own well-being for a few minutes in silence.

2. The next expansion of your field of metta is to someone known as "the benefactor," someone who has been good to you, has taken care of you, has been generous or inspiring; someone who reminds you of your own full capacity as a human being to be loving, compassionate, and aware. If there is such a person in your life or somebody comes to mind, you can either bring forth an image of that person, perhaps saying the person's name quietly to yourself, or picture that person's face in your mind's eye. Remember the good that person has done for you or the person's good qualities, and begin offering the person loving-kindness through the same phrases and intentions: *May you be free from danger*, *May you be happy*, *May you be healthy*, *May you live with ease*.

3. After a few minutes of focusing on the benefactor, open your heart further to include a friend or loved one. If you think of a loved one, you can visualize that person, say the person's name, bring the person into your heart in some sense, and include the person in the

power of this intention of friendship, of loving-kindness. See if you can extend to your loved one the same wish you extended to yourself: *May you be free from danger, May you be happy, May you be healthy, May you live with ease.*

4. The next person to extend loving-kindness to is the "neutral person." Someone for whom you don't have a strong like or dislike, maybe someone you encounter in the routine of day-to-day life. If you can think of such a person, remember that this person, like all beings everywhere, simply wants to be happy. You may not know the person well or understand the person's particular situation, but you do know this: that all beings everywhere want to be happy. So extend to this person the happiness, freedom, love, and joy you would wish for yourself or your loved ones.

5. You may wish to stop here, but if you'd like to move on, the next person is known as the "difficult person." Usually it's better at this point not to use the most difficult person in your life but, rather, someone who has troubled you in a mild or annoying way. Gradually, over time, you may find it in your heart to extend kindness even to a person who has had a part in causing you a great deal of suffering. Remember that when we offer friendship or loving-kindness, it's not in the sense of condoning someone's hurtful actions or about pretending we feel something other than what we actually feel. It's about recognizing our shared predicament of suffering, our connectedness as living beings existing together in this world.

6. We then turn to directing our sense of caring, of loving-kindness, to all beings everywhere: *May all beings be free from danger, May all beings be happy, May all beings be healthy,* and *May all beings live with ease.*

As you complete metta meditation, consider maintaining awareness of a sense of compassion toward yourself and other living beings as you go about your day and life. You may find that the sense of connectedness that metta practice cultivates brings about a qualitative difference in your interactions with others and provides an antidote to any tendencies you have toward selfishness or self-centeredness.

LOVING-KINDNESS MEDITATION FOR SELF-HEALING

You may already be familiar with the way we often distinguish between healing and cure. "Cure" typically refers to ridding the body of disease—in this case, becoming free of all signs of cancer. "Healing," on the other hand, is a holistic term that considers the well-being of the entire body, mind, and spirit, which are indivisible. It's possible for you to be cured of your cancer, but you are not completely healed if you still suffer from depression or worry or feel lost or disconnected in your life. Conversely, it's also possible for you to heal even if your cancer is not technically "cured." You may be living with cancer still in your body, with or without active symptoms, yet still be able to feel at peace. We hope you receive this quality of healing or sense of wholeness, whether or not you are medically cured. The loving-kindness meditation practice can be very helpful in your process of healing.

Susan, a woman in our program, found it very uncomfortable and felt it was selfish and inappropriate to sit around wishing for her own happiness. She saw this act as self-indulgent and herself as unworthy of this kind of attention. After all, she felt it was her own fault she was ill with cancer, and she now saw herself as simply paying the price. She was very harsh and demanding with herself, and although she had completed her leukemia treatment, she was not healed or even moving toward healing in the sense of the word as we conceptualize it. When she first did the metta meditation in the daylong retreat, she felt uncomfortable and angry. While many in the group immediately found it to be a healing practice, with several people even shedding tears, this was not the case for Susan.

In the next class, she mentioned her reservations about the practice and heard others' comments about their experiences. Surprised that so many people had found metta to be a calming, warm, and nurturing practice, she asked them, "Didn't you feel self-indulgent doing this?" Group members shared that in contrast, this meditation helped them to feel connected with others and as if they were giving back by sincerely wishing for their own and others' well-being and happiness. In a sense, they could feel that connection of common humanity and suffering as simply part of the human condition. By relaxing into their own wish for happiness and health, they could accept that their desire for happiness was no more selfish than all other beings' same wish for their own happiness.

The realization that we all are flawed and that we all suffer allows for a softening of rigid expectations for your own conduct that you may not apply to others. Susan was able to see and have compassion for others' suffering, but not her own. An element of self-compassion is an entryway to your healing process. Practicing metta can help to build this capacity simply by making you realize that your own happiness or suffering is no different from that of your friends, loved ones, and even enemies. Repeated practice will help you, first, to recognize your own suffering and, second, to allow yourself to accept wishes for healing and compassion, from both yourself and others.

HOW TO PRACTICE A DAY OF SILENCE

We suggest choosing a day that works for you after you have practiced the basic meditations and yoga for several weeks, and either practice alone or invite some friends who may also be interested or already involved in meditation practice. Plan a schedule for the day, as structured or unstructured as you like, and find an appropriate setting for your practice. A quiet, warm room with ample space and light or an outdoor setting would be nice. Make sure there won't be any interruptions and, of course, unplug or turn off your phones, laptops, and so forth. Prepare your materials in advance and, if you plan to use guided meditations, make sure you have recordings or DVDs ready. Also be sure to plan for some standing, walking, or stretching to break up periods of sitting. Prepare lunch in advance, or include lunch preparation as a meditation of its own. Most important, throughout the day, just bear in mind the idea of returning your attention to the present moment whenever it wanders, really focusing on maintaining your mindfulness throughout each practice.

You may want to practice more spontaneously, without a schedule, and just sit until you feel you have had enough and then walk, and so on. You may want to have inspiring music or include incense burning or aromatherapy. The possibilities are all up to you. Perhaps enjoy some poetry reading if that helps you connect with your practice. After the day of silence, try to ease your way back into your day to see if you can maintain some of the feelings from the practice as you move back into everyday interactions.

CHAPTER 10

Deepening and Expanding

The Guest House
This being human is a guest house,
Every morning a new arrival.
A joy, a depression, a meanness,
Some momentary awareness comes
As an unexpected visitor.
Welcome and entertain them all!
Even if they're a crowd of sorrows,
Who violently sweep your house
Empty of its furniture.
Still, treat each guest honorably.
They may be clearing you out
For some new delight.
The dark thought, the shame, the malice,
Meet them at the door laughing,
And invite them in.
Be grateful for whoever comes,
Because each has been sent
As a guide from beyond.

—Rumi (in *A Year with Rumi*, 366)

If you have made it this far in the book and have practiced what you have read, you will likely have experienced periods of peacefulness, stability, and equanimity in your practice. You will have developed some capacity to concentrate and intentionally sustain awareness of bodily sensations, the breath, sensory experience, thought, and emotion. We have guided you through these practices in a stepwise fashion, and you may have begun to appreciate how the sense of self is woven from these strands of experience.

Next we will present an approach that might be best described as bare awareness of being, sometimes called "open awareness" or "choiceless awareness." In choiceless awareness meditation, you sit in the middle of experience and remain attentive and open to whatever arises, without fear or favor. You don't seek any particular kind of experience; nor do you turn away from whatever comes up. You refrain from analyzing, judging, or evaluating, and from considering whatever arises in relation to yourself or your stories. You simply remain present, open, and receptive as being unfolds in your awareness. Initially, the most accessible way to begin choiceless-awareness practice probably is as an extension of sitting meditation; however, you can practice it anywhere, anytime, and in any body position.

PRACTICE 10.1
Choiceless Awareness

Take your seat. Sit comfortably, in a balanced and open posture with your spine erect. Breathe naturally. Check in. Begin to attend to your body with awareness and an attitude of hospitality that welcomes whatever presents itself.

Now settled in, with attention stabilized in body awareness—shifting focus for a while to awareness of breathing—in a similar manner, proceeding to check in with the other sensory channels—as if sampling or registering awareness of the emerging present through each mode of perception—the world of experience manifesting as vibrations of various frequencies, and the senses' gateways—intentionally, awareness of vision, sound, smell, taste, emotion, and thought each holding center stage for a time—as much as possible, being aware of what emerges as bare sensation, without naming, identifying, or interpreting—yet noticing any tendency to analyze in this way and letting go of it as it occurs.

At some point, letting go of any specific intentional focus and establishing a more even, open, receptive stance toward whatever is arising—becoming an equal opportunity perceiver—with no right or wrong aspect of experience to notice—noticing whatever arises in the forefront of awareness without succumbing to the need to elaborate, act, or judge—as surely as night follows day, other aspects of experience will move to the fore, supplanting what was there—allowing all of it to play out within the vastness of awareness—from time to time, perhaps discovering attachment to some aspect of experience and noticing lost mindfulness—this is okay—stepping back, beginning again right here and now—regaining mindfulness—which may happen repeatedly—if it occurs too frequently, perhaps reestablishing concentration by sitting with full awareness of breathing for a while and returning to choiceless awareness at some other time.

CHOICELESS AWARENESS AS A PATH OF INSIGHT

The moments when, as described in the choiceless-awareness meditation instructions, you can step out of the prisonlike view of self-referential thought and experience—these moments reveal truths about your existence that are obscured when you are trapped in the conditioning of your habits, worries, and problems.

The moments when you realize the "suchness" of things as they are—that is, their bare-bones nature, undefiled by concepts—allow you to touch the fundamental beauty of your existence. You also see that the phenomenal world is ever changing, fragile, and marked by impermanence. This realization can alarm you as your stable sense of self as solid and enduring is threatened; it can also liberate you if you can practice letting go of the ties that bind you to the illusion of your separateness. In its place, the vehicle of choiceless awareness gives you glimpses of wholeness.

CHOICELESS AWARENESS AND CANCER

Of course, for anyone living with a cancer diagnosis, thoughts and fears about the future can be almost constant companions, aspects of conditioning that may hold near trancelike sway over day-to-day life. This is especially true if troublesome symptoms provide frequent reminders of illness.

Julia, a patient of ours living with metastatic breast cancer, shared some of her thoughts about this. She spoke of the advice others (usually people without cancer) had often given her to "live for today," and how difficult that was for her to even contemplate. As much sense as it made to her intellectually, it wasn't easy for her to escape thoughts that plagued her about the future, which often centered around fears of leaving her young children without a mother to care for them and see them through to adolescence and adulthood.

For Julia, mindfulness practice, especially choiceless awareness, proved to be pivotal. Choiceless awareness meditation was where Julia could first begin to remain present with her fears while relating to them differently from the way she usually did. Initially, she had virtually wrestled with these thoughts, trying to push them out of awareness or avoid thinking about them altogether. Paradoxically perhaps, the net effect of this process had been to strengthen the hold her fears had on her consciousness. Julia had organized herself around resistance to these fears, and partly because of this, they persisted, standing firmly at center stage.

In her mindfulness practice, Julia intentionally began working with the possibility of simply remaining present with these thoughts as they emerged, without engaging them in any way. Without resisting or avoiding, she cultivated equanimity, aided by awareness of the steady flow of her breath. In the absence of resistance, she found room for other kinds of experiences to emerge. She was able to experience her fear-producing thoughts as well as moments of calm. The unsettling uncertainty of cancer was sometimes apparent, yet also available to her was the feeling of being grounded in the sensations of her own body as it sat restfully moment by moment. She became poignantly aware of the preciousness of the people and things she loved in this world, and the fact that they were available to her in her daily life right now!

All of this and more visited her over time, and this mindfulness practice helped her develop a view of the fullness of her life without letting cancer dominate the picture. Julia felt that directly facing the enormity of her situation was key to really being able to live more often by the advice others had given so easily: live each day to its fullest. Despite her having concluded, "Much easier said than done," her determined choice to open to the full range of her experience had allowed her to find a way that felt right for her.

CHAPTER 11

Moving into the World

Seas

I have a feeling that my boat

Has struck, down there in the depths,

Against a great thing.

And nothing

Happens! Nothing...silence...waves.

Nothing happens? Or has everything happened,

And are we standing now, quietly, in the new life?

—Juan Ramón Jiménez

Whether initially you felt some doubt or reluctance or you felt genuine enthusiasm, we hope that you were able to dive into this book with a sense of curiosity and good intentions and that you have already begun your journey to mindfulness. If you've done so, you have likely learned a great deal about mindfulness and about yourself in the process. Maybe you have attended a class, workshop, or retreat for some concentrated practice, and really feel that mindfulness is making a difference in your life. Now what's next? Many on-and-off meditators can attest that without some sort of plan, there's a real risk your budding practice will wither on the vine.

YOU ARE NOT ALONE

If you practice mindfulness all alone out in the wide world, it can be very difficult to sustain your practice amid the chaos and countervailing influences of modern life. Many competing interests virtually demand your attention, and excessive duties and responsibilities can threaten to undermine your good intentions.

One measure that will help you sustain your practice is to find or develop a mindfulness community. It's heartening to realize that there are millions of meditators around the world. Consider that at this very moment, somewhere in the world, people, maybe hundreds of people, are practicing loving-kindness meditation and sending wishes for your well-being. It's wonderful to realize that when you sit in mindfulness or practice loving-kindness meditation, many others are also doing so.

In nearly every community live people just like you, who aim to live ethical and mindful lives; if you are fortunate, you can find a group that meets regularly to learn and practice. A meditation center or yoga studio may be nearby, where you can meet other practitioners and discover opportunities to sit. We know of small groups of friends that get together informally to practice and perhaps to share a cup of tea and conversation afterward. In taking it upon herself to organize a major retreat, one woman who completed our eight-week course brought a celebrated teacher to town and thus made many new connections.

Many larger population centers have Buddhist congregations that often offer opportunities for newcomers to learn meditation and Buddhist dharma or teachings. You don't have to give up your own faith tradition and won't be expected to do so. There are many meditation traditions and techniques, and it's really up to you to find a practice context that's right for you. Some trial and error may be required to find a good fit.

Look for ways to bring mindfulness to your doorstep and Internet browser. Many fine publications and websites focus on the wisdom traditions, which can expand your horizons and provide steady reminders to practice, so we have listed some of them in the appendix to help you get started.

THE WEEKLY DROP-IN GROUP

To give you an example of how enriching and supportive a mindfulness-practice community can be, we'll tell you the story of a very special community we have been a part of. At our cancer treatment center every Thursday afternoon since 1999, a wonderful collection of "fortunate friends" has come together for a period of practice, sharing, and supportive interaction. These men and women have two things in common: all have been diagnosed with cancer and completed our eight-week MBCR program at some point during their journey.

Each week the format remains the same. After an initial period of meditation, we pass the meditation bells around the circle, and, punctuated by the bells' sounding, all present are invited to share something about their lives, illness, and practice; however they choose to use that time is up to each of them. What they share is the stuff of life, big and small, often with observations about the role their practice has played in coloring their experience. At times it's an occasion for profound sharing and other times for humor, but fundamentally it's a way of connecting at a very basic human level and of supporting each other.

We then move together through some yoga asanas and finish with a period of meditation practice. The form of practice varies. Though we often sit together in silent practice, on a lovely spring day, we might find ourselves outside walking the banks of the nearby river, where we breathe the fresh air; hear the flowing water; and feel the earth beneath our feet, the wind in our faces, and the sun's warmth on our skin. We invite people to bring to the group questions about other contemplative practices they have experienced or participated in, and we are open to suggestions for new meditation practices they would like to familiarize themselves with. We have had guest teachers who have introduced the group to qigong, a form of Chinese meditation and breath work, and tai chi, a type of moving meditation many are now familiar with.

The group also supports one another through difficult times. When one woman had grown ill from her cancer's progression and could no longer attend the group, we made a recording of each group member

145

reading a passage of a guided healing meditation. We worked together on the script, and group members chose the material they wanted to include on the recording and which sections they wanted to read. A close friend delivered the resulting CD to the woman at home. She let us know that the recording helped comfort and calm her when she couldn't make it to the group in person. She listened to that recording regularly until her eventual death from metastatic cancer. Many group members attended her funeral.

As we saw this group grow over the years, we became interested in studying it in more depth, because we could see a phenomenon happening there that was not evident in the initial eight-week group we had studied up to that point. To do this, we conducted a simple interview study with seven longtime group members (Mackenzie et al. 2007), simply asking them why they kept coming week after week to meditate together. What we learned was quite profound. Their stories helped us see a process of development that had happened for them over the years. At first, meeting together for practice helped them radically shift their views of how to cope with life situations. They learned about letting go of the illusion of control and being mindfully in the moment, which helped them deal more easily with the demands of cancer treatment that most were dealing with when they first took the program. They realized in hindsight that the eight-week group had been just the tip of the iceberg. They told us that their most profound changes had taken place since that time, as they continued to practice week after week and year after year.

The lessons that came early in the practice were how to self-regulate emotional reactions and respond mindfully, rather than react automatically, to stressful life situations. After that, in addition to continuing to help in that area, the practice enabled them to grow and transform as individuals, emphasizing feelings of gratitude and helping them develop compassion for others over time. They described feeling more connected with others in their lives and continually realizing the value of slowing down and enjoying connecting with nature.

An interesting topic that came up was how the meditation practice helped strengthen their sense of spirituality. By that, they weren't referring to religiosity, which generally describes participation in a particular religious tradition and its accompanying rituals. Rather, spirituality

146

refers to a felt sense of connection with something larger than yourself, often encompassing issues of where you find meaning and purpose in life. Despite the deliberate absence of planned discussion of spirituality and religion in MBCR groups, this element emerged spontaneously over time for most people we talked to.

Another extremely important part of group attendance for these people was the support of the group itself, for not only practicing meditation but also connecting with other cancer survivors who had been through similar experiences. Although the cancer journey wasn't regularly discussed in the drop-in group, just the awareness of this shared adversity helped the group cohere over time. One of the participants summed up this sentiment:

> That's what is really special about the group, hearing about
> what people are coping with. You can listen to someone talk
> about their suffering, and you can accommodate that. You
> don't have to walk away from it. I was pretty good at doing
> that before I went through this whole thing.... I'm really happy
> I have an opportunity to know about those things.... You don't
> want to run from that. (Mackenzie et al. 2007, 64)

PART III

Symptom Management and Everyday Mindfulness

CHAPTER 12

Mindful Coping with Cancer-Related Symptoms and Side Effects

I said to the wanting-creature inside me:
What is this river you want to cross?
There are no travelers on the river-road, and no road.
Do you see anyone moving about on that bank, or resting?
There is no river at all, and no boat, and no boatman.
There is no towrope either, and no one to pull it.
There is no ground, no sky, no time to bank, no ford!
And there is no body, and no mind!
Do you believe there is some place that will make the soul less thirsty?
In that great absence you will find nothing.

Be strong then, and enter into your own body;
There you have a solid place for your feet.
Think about it carefully!
Don't go off somewhere else!
Just throw away all thoughts of imaginary things,
And stand firm in that which you are.

—Kabir

Dealing with cancer involves more than worry and stress about the illness itself, the treatments, and the prognosis for the future. The very real and troubling physical symptoms of disease and side effects of treatment also cause great upset and suffering. Such disturbances range from the most obvious outward marker of cancer for many patients—hair loss—to inner changes, such as an altered self-image and problems with energy levels, including profound fatigue and difficulty sleeping that can turn into a vicious circle of sleepless nights, tired days, daytime napping, and more sleepless nights.

Cancer patients often also encounter many types of pain, from painful procedures like biopsies, blood draws, chemotherapy administration, and radiation therapy to postsurgical pain and lingering aches and pains from the illness itself. The practices you have learned in this book specifically apply to all of these problems, plus they generally help reduce your stress and improve your overall quality of life. Note that being in distress initiates excitatory and inflammatory responses that can exacerbate many side effects, but good evidence shows that relaxation alone can reduce the intensity of such side effects (Sloman 1995).

HAIR LOSS AND CHANGES IN SELF-IMAGE AND IDENTITY

Often one of the most difficult side effects of many types of chemotherapy is hair loss. Many people see this as the official "badge" of the cancer patient. Hair loss makes it difficult to hide the illness from others or to deny that it's really happening—even to yourself if you are the one with cancer. People in general are very attached to their hair. It's part of what makes you recognizable as yourself. You might describe yourself as a redhead or blond, with characteristic short or long hair that's straight or curly, and this may be a central part of your identity. You might not even realize the importance you place on your hair until it begins to fall right out in clumps, you have to clear the shower drain, or you don't even recognize yourself in the mirror anymore. Who is this person staring back at you with the funny-looking baldhead? As an indisputable symbol of loss, it can trigger a deep sense of grief. Friends and acquaintances may pass you by, failing to recognize you and making you start to wonder, *Who am I anyway?*

Women are sometimes mistaken for men, when this outward sign of femininity is taken away, and as sometimes occurs, your school-age children may feel uncomfortable being seen with you in public when you're not wearing a wig or they may stop asking their friends to your home. *Am I now just a generic "cancer patient" and that's all anyone sees?* This fundamental shift in appearance can make you question other aspects of your identity as well. *Am I still the mother, father, carpenter, lawyer, or administrative assistant I used to be? What is it that really makes me* me, *and how can I get that back?* The following meditation is a way for you to examine the fundamental questions of who you are that self-image challenges integral to the cancer experience may bring up.

PRACTICE 12.1
Who Are You?

Take a comfortable seat where you can sit balanced and upright, and breathe easily. Take a moment to tune in to your breath as it flows in and out of your body. Feel its rhythm. Begin to feel your body as a whole, pulsating with each breath in and out. After a few moments, when you feel settled into the rhythm of the breath, begin to pose a series of silent questions to yourself. These may begin with the most peripheral aspects of yourself, such as your possessions: *Am I what I possess? Am I defined by my car, my house, my clothes, my shoes? Are these things what make me* me?

You may not have ready answers to any of these questions; what's important is simply to pose them to yourself and allow yourself time to breathe and sit with each question. Then ask yourself, *If I am not these things, then what am I?* Again, there's no ready answer to this question. Just try to sit and breathe with the question.

Perhaps then move on to aspects of yourself that you may be more attached to: *Am I what I do? Am I defined by the roles I play in life? Am I a mother, a daughter, a son, a sibling, my occupation, a cancer patient or survivor?* If you didn't have these roles to play, what or who would you be then?

Am I defined by my personal characteristics, such as my personality or my likes and dislikes? Do I define myself by my talents? Am I a singer, a dancer, a reader, a writer? A cheerful person, a cynic, a dog lover? Are these the things that make me me? *What if all these things were lost too? Who would I be then?*

Am I this physical body? Is this body sitting here the same as the one I was born with? What makes me feel that it is, when nothing is the same as when I was born? What if my body radically changed? If I lost my sight, my hair, my ability to walk or run, would I still be me?

Am I my mind, my thoughts? Those never-ending thoughts that rise and fall constantly in my conscious mind—do those define who I am?

What if all of this were stripped away? What would I be? Would I still be me?

Still sitting and breathing quietly, consider the possibility that you are none of these things. Is it possible that you could be more vast, that your essence could be other than any connection to the body you now reside in, the thoughts you harbor, your likes or dislikes, your talents or roles in life? What might that feel like?

Can your identity really be known without a sense of who you were before you were born and who you will be after you die? And can your identity really be known in isolation, disconnected from your friends, family, society, and environment?

Could it be that what's essential about you transcends your ideas and beliefs about yourself and involves your connection to a larger web of being and becoming, a web that connects you with all beings coexisting in the vastness of time, the web of life?

This may not make sense to you, but that's okay. Just continue to sit for a few minutes more with the possibility that you are something beyond any material or personal characteristics you possess, things that change day to day and year to year; the possibility that you, your consciousness, is part of a more encompassing and enduring form of awareness.

The intent of the previous practice is to help you begin to see that the traditional things you may consider important in defining your place in the world are often transitory. There's a more stable and enduring dimension to your being, and connecting with this possibility through your meditation practice may help soothe the pain of changes to your self-image and identity that cancer triggers.

SLEEP AND FATIGUE

Another troubling side effect for many people living with cancer, not only cancer patients but also their family members, is difficulty sleeping well and always feeling tired. For the cancer patient, fatigue is often the result of cancer and its treatments. You may have trouble sleeping for many reasons: the anxiety and worry of the whole process, an upset in your usual schedule, sleeping in different locations, physiological arousal due to stimulating medications you may have to take, effects of chemotherapy drugs, changes in your exercise or physical activity regimen, altered eating patterns, and the list could go on. In fact, research shows that up to 80 percent of cancer patients have sleep problems during treatment, and up to half still have these problems well after treatment completion (Savard and Morin 2001).

We published a study that asked approximately sixty patients going through the MBCR program about their sleep patterns both before and after the program (Carlson and Garland 2005). The questionnaire we used asked very detailed questions about several aspects of sleep, such as how quickly people fell asleep once they went to bed, how long they slept, how often they woke up during the night, how they felt in the morning, their use of sleeping medications, and more. What we found was quite striking: on average, people reported sleeping up to an hour more each night after the program, and they subjectively felt that they were sleeping much better. They also reported fewer stress symptoms and felt less fatigued. We also looked at the associations between improvements in sleep and changes in mood, stress, and fatigue levels. Not surprisingly, when people showed decreases in their stress levels, they also slept better and had more energy.

Here's a handy sleep practice you can use anytime you're in bed and having difficulty sleeping. It incorporates several principles and techniques you learned in chapter 6 on breathing: first, switch to a nice, deep belly breath, and then control your breathing rate so that you are breathing out for twice the count that you breathe in; this is called a "two-to-one" breath. For example, if you breathe in for a count of four, then try to modulate your outbreath so that you slowly breathe out for a count of eight. To do this, you will need to breathe out a smaller volume, as if you are breathing out through a straw. Once you get the hang of the two-to-one breath, add another element based on the theory behind alternate-nostril breathing.

Begin by lying neutrally on your back, but then switch to your left side, which opens up your right nostril (and the more active part of your brain), and then finish off by lying on your right side, which opens up your left nostril, putting you in a relaxed, receptive state of mind that's ideal for sleep. This practice is great because it not only evokes the physiology you need for sleep but also distracts your racing mind with counting so you are focused on the present moment rather than lying there worrying, ruminating, or planning. Together, these conditions create the ideal setting for a good night's sleep.

PRACTICE 12.2
Sleep Practice

1. Get into bed and pay close attention to your breath:

   a. Allow the breath to become smooth and deep.

   b. Eliminate the pause between inhalation and exhalation.

   c. Switch to a two-to-one breathing pattern (breathing out for twice the time you breathe in).

2. Follow this sequence for number of breaths and positions:

   a. Take eight breaths while lying on your back.

   b. Take sixteen breaths while lying on your left side.

   c. Take thirty-two breaths while lying on your right side.

3. Repeat the entire sequence if you are still awake.

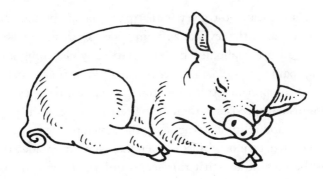

A good night's sleep is also the first step in reducing any fatigue you may be experiencing. Another great treatment for fatigue is exercise; the yoga postures we taught you in chapter 5 will help reduce fatigue if you practice them daily. We also suggest fresh air and regular walks as soon as you are up to it. We recommend thirty minutes of mild to moderate exercise a day for people who have been through cancer, to help lessen fatigue and improve quality of life.

PAIN

Cancer patients often experience pain in a variety of situations, and it can crop up virtually anytime. One way to begin working with pain is to invite relaxation through balanced abdominal breathing. As mentioned previously, being in distress initiates excitatory and inflammatory responses that can increase pain. Deep relaxation alone can reduce the perceived intensity of pain (Sloman 1995).

When you have settled in to relative comfort, bring your awareness to the painful area in your body, just as you would for a body scan. At first, this might seem counterintuitive and your pain might seem worse, but stick with it for a moment. You may notice some clenching or tightening of the muscles around the pain, a general holding or protection of the area. This tension can cause the pain to escalate and increase your level of suffering. Attempting to wall off or block pain from your awareness is often counterproductive. Here's a helpful equation:

$$\text{Suffering} = \text{Pain} \times \text{Resistance}$$

What this is meant to convey is that pain may be present, but your resistance to it makes the level of suffering you experience much worse.

This resistance is embodied by both physically clenching and mentally pushing pain away. A large part of what's known as "total pain" is the emotional component. At the emotional level, resistance can take the form of anguished, persistent thought patterns and resentment. At the level of thought and attitude, rather than the actual pain experienced in a given moment, what's most difficult to endure is often the idea that pain will always be present and that this seems unfair. If you can shift your emotional reactions to pain—for example, by approaching the sensations in your awareness with a sense of curiosity, openness, and acceptance—resistance and suffering often diminish.

After bringing awareness to the painful area, sense any holding or resistance around it; breathing slowly and deeply, see if you can release the muscular tension in the surrounding area. For some people, imagining the breath or warm energy moving into the area facilitates release. Now instead of avoiding the pain sensations, take the opportunity to investigate the pain more intimately. What are its actual contours? Does it have a shape? Are its boundaries rigid or moving? Is it constant or varying in intensity? Does it change over time or with positional shifts? One way to think about this is to learn to relate to the actual sensations we call pain so that what once seemed solid and unchanging takes on a more fluid and shifting quality. Integrating the sensations within a broader context of awareness can allow some dis-identification and spaciousness around the experience of pain that can soften the harshness of the pain experience.

This is not a simple process, and there are entire books that tackle the issue of pain control with the use of meditation. Jon Kabat-Zinn's *Full Catastrophe Living* (Delacorte Press, 1990) is a useful reference, as is *The Mindfulness Solution to Pain*, by Jackie Gardner-Nix with Lucie Costin-Hall (New Harbinger Publications, 2009).

In research Kabat-Zinn's team did with people experiencing chronic pain, they found that although pain levels themselves did not decrease a whole lot over time (note that these people had enduring chronic pain syndromes), what did change was the suffering the pain caused (Kabat-Zinn, Lipworth, and Burney 1985; Kabat-Zinn et al. 1986). The people who went through the MBSR program were better able to relate to their pain, soften around it, and see it as a shifting, porous, and workable process. This stance toward pain made all the difference in the world to study participants and can mean real changes in terms of functioning and the possibility for enjoyment of life.

Sharon, a breast-cancer patient who took our program during the course of chemotherapy, was on a new regimen that included the addition of a medication to stimulate bone growth, but it caused her terrible bone pain in her back and legs. When she first learned the body scan and sitting meditations, she expressed that it was just so hard to focus on her breath or the specified body part when she was experiencing such intense pain. Another woman in the group, Lorraine, shared that she, too, was on that same regimen and also had terrible bone pain during her meditation but somehow was able to shift her attention to the painful area, focus on that area, and relax the muscles, leading to a real reduction in her experience of the pain itself. A discussion ensued in which these women and several other participants shared instances when they were able to change the way they related to their pain by paying attention to it in a different way. They said that though the meditation didn't completely eliminate the pain, it somehow made it more tolerable. They recognized that it was often the thoughts they had about the pain that made it seem unbearable.

NAUSEA

The same goes for other unpleasant sensations, such as nausea. Nausea may be the inevitable consequence of a number of cancer treatments, although the recent generation of antinausea drugs is so good that we don't encounter this problem as much as we used to. However, tension and worry about the possibility of nausea definitely make it worse. Deep breathing and relaxation can help to alleviate nausea, and meditation practice can help you to accept it as the way things are in the moment.

Another, related problem some people experience is *anticipatory nausea*, a learned response that can happen if a certain procedure or treatment caused you nausea in the past. For example, John, a lymphoma patient in our program, had a strong reaction to his chemotherapy drugs and experienced quite severe nausea and vomiting after his first treatment. The antinausea drug they gave him didn't work so well, but they eventually found a better one. However, the memory of that first experience was so strongly imprinted that John began to experience nausea while just driving into the cancer-center parking lot. The sensation got worse as he walked in the door and headed to the chemotherapy area, to the point where he had to run to the bathroom several times and almost vomited.

All of this happened without his being exposed to any drugs at all; it was the product of his mind and the strong aversive conditioning of that first bad experience. That's why having an effective antinausea protocol from the start is a good idea. You can also use the techniques we've introduced to help control this kind of nausea. Several studies have investigated this possibility and found very positive results (see, for example, Carey and Burish 1987). Try using the script in practice 12.3 if you ever experience anticipatory reactions to your treatment.

PRACTICE 12.3
Reducing Anticipatory Nausea

First, find a comfortable seat where you can hold yourself upright with ease and breathe fully and deeply. Take a few moments to connect with the breath, allowing it to slow and deepen without forcing it; just relax naturally. Notice any tension in the body: the eyes, the jaw, the shoulders, or any other place where you typically hold tension. Allow it to melt away as you exhale. Spend a few minutes just settling into this place of silence: imagine yourself as a silty glass of water; just sit and allow the particles to settle to the bottom and the water to become clear. Only time and patience can allow this to happen.

When you feel clear and settled, imagine the situation that typically brings on the swell of nausea, maybe the sight of the treatment center or entering the building. Pause there when you first realize the nausea's beginnings. Notice the surroundings and smells you imagine, and notice the feelings in your body. It's okay if you feel a little of the nausea; now you can just focus on the breath once again and allow it to pass. Just breathe in and out, feeling the belly rising and falling gently. Let your muscles become smooth and relaxed. Allow yourself to remain in this imaginary place for as long as you need to, until you feel comfortable enough to move on. When you are ready, imagine yourself moving closer to the destination, the place or event that usually leads to feeling sick. At each step of the way, check in with yourself, and if you begin to feel overwhelmed, stop and take however long you need to get back to that comfortable, settled feeling you had earlier. It may help to generate an antinausea image to supplant the thoughts that trigger your discomfort. This could be a fond picture or memory; the sound of your favorite music; the fragrance of fresh, clean air on a pleasant summer day; or even a warm, vibrant color that makes you feel wonderful when you see it. Skiing is a very popular pastime in our area, and several of our patients have used the image of cool mountain air and snow flurries settling on and quelling the turbulence in the stomach.

Eventually, stopping when necessary, imagine yourself completing the entire activity that has become associated with uncomfortable feelings for you. Allow yourself to do this in your mind's eye, while maintaining a calm and focused presence in the body as you continue to sit in this formal meditation.

After you have visualized yourself completing the activity, return your focus to simply the breath and body, feeling the gentle rise and fall of the breath with each inflow and outflow. When you are ready, open your eyes and return to your day.

Once you have done this meditation several times and can imagine yourself going through the entire scenario without experiencing the nausea, you may develop enough confidence to apply it to the real world. In the same way as in the meditation, apply the deep breathing and calming or soothing imagery to help you at each step of the way. Take your time as you approach the setting that has caused you trouble, and don't worry if it takes some practice.

CHAPTER 13

Knowing Your Fear and Other Difficult Emotions

It is not hard to live through a day if you can live through a moment. What creates despair is the imagination, which pretends there is a future and insists on predicting millions of moments, thousands of days, and so drains you that you cannot live the moment at hand.

—Andre Dubus

Fear, grief, and anger—as well as their cousins: anxiety, sadness, and frustration—are sometimes described as negative emotions. We're not so sure that's a helpful way of thinking about them. Though they seem to be an unwelcome and inevitable part of the illness experience, these difficult emotions can serve to help you learn and grow. Healing from emotional pain is at the heart of your growth as a complete human being. In fact, without coming to terms with these "darker" emotions in your life, healing may not be possible. In the face of adversity is really where you can discover your true strength. Fear, in particular, can be a near-constant companion in the dominion of cancer. From that moment when the words are spoken, "You have cancer," the solid feeling of the ground beneath your feet evaporates, your heart feels as if it's being crushed in your chest, and a sense of dread fills the pit of your stomach. The feeling may subside from time to time, but it stands close at hand, ready to cast its dark shadow at the slightest provocation. A twinge of pain somewhere in the body, the oppressive wait for a test result, or a friend or physician's poorly chosen word is all it may take to rouse that sense of foreboding and fear.

THE PARADOX OF AVOIDANCE

Not surprisingly, people often do anything they can to escape such unpleasant feelings; for some threats, running away is exactly what's called for. In the case of cancer-related fears and emotional pain, there really is no place to run and hide. Instead, you may substitute psychological defense mechanisms, like avoidance or repression, which are tricks we humans use to keep fear away from our center of awareness and which can provide a temporary reprieve.

Unfortunately, the painful emotions don't just go away; they lie in wait, ready to pounce as perceived threat mounts, losses accumulate, or your defenses become exhausted. In fact, avoidance of painful emotions actually reinforces and increases their power over you. What does it say when you treat a danger as so threatening you can't even acknowledge it?

OPENING TO EMOTIONAL SUFFERING

One of the most powerful tools for working with fear and other emotions is to turn to face their source, rather than turn away. When Dorothy and her companions are trembling in the presence of the fearsome Wizard of Oz, they are instructed to avoid by ignoring the man behind the curtain. But in the clarity of that moment, they do see the true nature of the source of their fear: it's no wizard at all, just a man. So it often is with cancer-related fears and other emotions: the imagined is far more threatening than the reality. Rather than destroy you, your emotions can guide you to your strengths. What you require is a context that enables you to face your emotions openly.

Well-run cancer support groups serve just such a purpose, and your meditation practice can similarly provide a crucible for relating to your emotional life from a place of relative safety. Within the vastness that is awareness, you can hold, acknowledge, and honor the emotions you experience, yet recognize that you are not your emotions. There's much more to you, including awareness itself, which is not afraid, sad, or angry. One advantage of this type of process is that openly acknowledging your fears allows practical and effective resources to be brought to bear to deal with their underlying sources.

Earlier we mentioned two kinds of coping: problem focused and emotion focused. Emotions often point the way toward problems that actually do have practical solutions amenable to problem-focused coping. When we broach the subject of fears, patients often say it's not death itself they fear, but the process of dying and the possibility of suffering specific outcomes, such as pain, breathlessness, and dependency. Identifying these fears makes it possible to talk about them with your physicians and others you trust. You can correct myths and misperceptions through that process and learn more about how to effectively manage challenges. Other fears and emotions are better dealt with using emotion-focused strategies, such as meditation.

WORKING WITH DIFFICULT EMOTIONS

In your meditation practice, you may encounter fear and other emotional pain as part of your experience. Fortunately, you can also discover the strength and courage necessary to remain present and respond in meaningful ways. It has been commonly observed that courage is not the absence of fear but, rather, choosing to respond skillfully in its presence.

Your first task as a mindfulness practitioner is to greet a painful emotion as it arises, and know it directly. You can recognize and acknowledge the fear. You can hold it in awareness and take a step back so you can see it as an element of your experience rather than your totality. Along with fear, you can also recognize your capacity to remain steady, breathe, and feel the ebb and flow of sensation, which may include fear as well as other sensations. You will see that you are not your fear, grief, or anger.

CALMING THE ANXIOUS MIND

During a first MBCR class we led recently, a man named David described his fears this way: "It gets so bad I even find myself picking out my casket." He wasn't someone who was imminently dying; in fact he had completed treatments for skin cancer, and all he could do now was wait and hope it didn't come back. This waiting with nothing concrete to do was torture for him, an active go-getter who just wanted to *do* something.

David realized, though, that in this case the best thing to do was nothing, to let go of these spiraling thoughts and anxieties he had no control over. That was why he was there in that class. We could see that it would be difficult for David at first, because he would have to sit quietly and listen to pounding anxieties going around and around in his mind, when all he wanted was to make them go away. Unfortunately, thoughts don't work like that; it's like saying to yourself *I must relax!* while tensing all your muscles—it's impossible. That's the paradox of meditation.

The only way David was going to achieve the quiet, peaceful mind he so desired was to let go of that straining and striving and just let his thoughts be, as unwanted as they were—open up the field of awareness to contain them and recognize that he need not react to them. He could instead remember to simply return his attention to his breath and other aspects of his experience in that moment, to witness the totality of his experience rather than remain captivated by the trance of his fears. In a way, worrying is a habit, and every time we react to worry by engaging with it, we reinforce or feed the habit. Choosing to simply rest in the presence of worry cuts it off from its primary source of energy, which is your reactiveness.

We often use analogies and metaphors as a means to explain some aspect of mindfulness practice. For example, you can experience problems, worries, and random thoughts in meditation as clouds that float across a clear, blue sky. Some days, the sky may be crowded with clouds; they may be little fluffy clouds or dark thunderheads. Some days may be relatively clear or just a little hazy. Just as you can't control the weather, you can't really control the clouds of thought. They arise, pass through, and disappear. It doesn't matter whether they are big and dark or light and fluffy thoughts. In fact thoughts are simply thoughts. They are, by no means, *the truth* about anything, so you don't need to react to them or try to suppress them. They are simply mind events, what the mind does if left idle.

Just having a thought that you forgot to turn off the porch light doesn't mean you have to immediately jump up, rush home, and turn it off. It might not even be true, and so what if it is? Your next thought might be that you'd like spaghetti for dinner or that the car needs a wash. Maybe so, but right now you can choose to attend to your breath. Many of these thoughts are just random clutter from your mind; accept them for what they are and carry on.

You might find yourself feeling very restless and wanting to get on with your day or writing to-do lists in your mind. Recognize that all those things can wait; they will still be there waiting for you when and if it's time to act on them. For this moment, however, be still, rest, and return to the breath; don't miss this moment for some other destination. Savor this moment, let go of the distracting thoughts, and return to being present with the sensations of breath and body, beginning anew each time your mind recognizes its own excursions. Instead of giving in to a sense of failure when you notice that your mind is wandering, accept it as inevitable and give yourself a mental pat on the back for noticing. Then simply begin again. Eventually you will learn that thoughts are just thoughts, whether they seem urgent or not; they are just blips your mind creates, not who you are. You are the endless blue sky beyond the thoughts; you are much more vast and constant than any passing thought, and you are still and deep and clear.

ANTIDOTES TO DIFFICULT EMOTIONS

One way to respond in the presence of difficult emotions is to call on other strengths and qualities to which you have access that you can further develop and strengthen. Loving-kindness practice, for example, can serve as an antidote to fear. The heart is often understood as the home of courage, and connecting to loving-kindness allows you to access what's most meaningful to you, which in turn strengthens your purpose and resolve.

Trust is also a powerful antidote to fear. There are different sources of trust in your life. Discovering that you can be present with your fear without being destroyed by it develops a kind of self-trust. Discovering that you can remain present and find a way to relate to whatever arises without being destroyed or consumed by it also strengthens this trust.

Another flavor of trust comes from a willingness to trust life itself, to trust the wisdom that created the world and gave you life and consciousness, by whatever name you know it. Fear is an emotion largely in service of preserving the ego, the created sense of self around which people build their lives. What happens if we trust in something much bigger than ourselves, if we open to a wider understanding of who we are, if we throw off the illusion of a separate and permanent self and willingly realize our place in the mystery of life and creation? In meditation we can ask ourselves, *Who am I really?* This may be the greatest act of courage and wisdom available to us.

CHAPTER 14

What Now?

The Summer Day
Who made the world?
Who made the swan, and the black bear?
Who made the grasshopper?
This grasshopper, I mean—
the one who has flung herself out of the grass,
the one who is eating sugar out of my hand,
who is moving her jaws back and forth instead of up and down—
who is gazing around with her enormous and complicated eyes.
Now she lifts her pale forearms and thoroughly washes her face.
Now she snaps her wings open, and floats away.
I don't know exactly what a prayer is.
I do know how to pay attention, how to fall down
into the grass, how to kneel down in the grass,
how to be idle and blessed, how to stroll through the fields,
which is what I have been doing all day.
Tell me, what else should I have done?
Doesn't everything die at last, and too soon?
Tell me, what is it you plan to do
with your one wild and precious life?

—Mary Oliver (in *New and Selected Poems*, vol. 1, 94)

As we near the end of this book, you might be wondering, what now? We have discussed the importance of joining a community of practice to help maintain the skills you have learned and continue deepening your mindfulness practice. This question, *What now?* applies not only to what comes next in your mindfulness practice but also to living as a cancer survivor. The end of active treatment can be a difficult time for many people; your friends and family may expect you to return to the life you led before this life-altering experience, but you may not feel that this is the best or healthiest option. If your former life was a hectic pursuit of socially sanctioned success, as is the case for many people, you may not want to return to that kind of "normal."

Surely there will be aspects of your former life you have missed and look forward to reengaging in, but you may decide that others are better left behind. You may also feel alone or abandoned by the support team you had during your cancer care, if you've recently been discharged from the treatment center. You likely have fears or concerns about the possibility the cancer will come back, what you can do to prevent it, and what kind of surveillance is required on your part. We addressed how mindfulness practice can help with some of these fears in the last chapter. In this chapter we want to discuss how you can live a more mindful life on an everyday basis, and how mindfulness can help you move beyond your experience and identity as a cancer survivor into the larger world.

EVERYDAY MINDFULNESS

If you'll recall, back in chapter 4 we made the distinction between formal and informal mindfulness practice. Since then, we have continued to introduce you to a wide range of formal meditation practices throughout the book. Now is the time to consider how these practices may have impacted your everyday life and how they can continue to do so. This is your informal practice, otherwise known as the rest of your life! Everyday mindfulness can take the form of the mini meditation practices we outlined in chapter 6, or it can simply ooze out into every moment of your life as you begin to integrate more fully the attitudes of joy, openness, curiosity, and attentiveness we first introduced in chapter 3. This change in attitude may be the most enduring legacy of training in mindfulness that can continue to profoundly touch the way you live every aspect of your life.

The poem that opened this chapter, "The Summer Day," by Mary Oliver, is a perfect illustration of this fresh approach. It's a poem of possibilities, of embracing the simple things in life that often bring the most joy, a real application of beginner's mind to every moment of life. Of course, this is not an easy or trivial thing to do; habits of worrying and ruminating are strong. Continuation of formal practice is what will help strengthen your informal mindfulness. You can help to bring moments of mindfulness to your everyday life by using cues you frequently encounter to remind yourself to bring your attention to whatever your experience is in a given moment. For example, every time a phone rings, use that as a cue to take a deep breath, take stock of how your body feels (as a tension gauge, for example), and prepare to respond mindfully to the person on the line. At each red light when you are driving, do the same kind of check-in with yourself. When you are walking, if you notice that your mind is elsewhere, stand still until you can draw your attention back to the moment. If you find yourself feeling impatient and cutting someone off in conversation, once again take some grounding breaths and notice how your body responds.

Most of all, just be where you are and notice when your judging mind pops up suggesting you'd rather be elsewhere or having some other experience. The fact of the matter is that you are *not* elsewhere, doing something else; you are where you are. We turn away from life only at great cost to ourselves. As the title of one of Jon Kabat-Zinn's books so obviously states: *Wherever You Go, There You Are.* The challenge is to see if you can be where you are and be fully aware of your experience, pleasant or not. One of our favorite sayings goes: "It is what it is." It's pretty obvious, but if you think about it, how often do you try to make it into something *other* than what it is? What suffering does this inevitably cause? What illusions take the place of what is? You certainly may want to make changes in your life so you can find yourself in unpleasant situations less often, but in the meantime, if you do encounter them, can you be where you are, remain open to what the moment offers, and learn and grow from it? The alternative is to still be there but be miserable and resentful about it the whole time. It's really your choice and also your opportunity to accept responsibility for your part in creating the experience.

LIFE AS YOUR PRACTICE

Another way to fortify your mindfulness practice is to infuse your daily life with awareness and aspire to live every moment of your life mindfully and wholeheartedly. What if you were to remind yourself at every opportunity that the life you are living is a sacred blessing, in fact, miraculous?

On awakening each day, can you marvel at the wonder of a new dawn? How would it be if, each day, you committed to living as if each moment of life were precious and holy, a rare gift, like rainfall in the desert? We are surrounded with beauty if we can slow down enough to notice, if we can step out of our preoccupations and actually commit to seeing. How would it feel to be appropriately grateful for all you are given, rather than craving more or wanting something else, some other life than the one you have? What if you brought to every situation you encountered and each person you met the questions, "Can I be present?" and "How can I help?"

PRACTICE 14.1
Living Meditation

Creating and holding an intention to bring awareness and heartfelt appreciation to each element of experience while moving through the day—on awakening in the morning, stretching and breathing—becoming aware of the body and its capacity to sustain life—being grateful—expressing gratitude for the eyes, ears, hands, toes, and all the rest—being thankful—for this very moment and each one to follow, giving thanks—for the possibility of living this very day, being joyful—in each person encountered, seeing that person's goodness, beauty, and wisdom—recognizing in that person a reflection of yourself—being kind—attuning the senses to the beauty and wonder of the natural world—breathing it in—breathing it out—greeting the day with eyes of wonder and a ready heart.

BEYOND CANCER

We've talked about the distinction between being healed and being cured; our hope is that developing a mindfulness practice will support your process of healing and recovery from your experience with cancer, whether you were the one with the illness or you were a support person. Healing is independent of cure; you may be living with cancer still in your body, or perhaps you are concerned that it may return. Despite this circumstance, you can still experience healing.

We mentioned our drop-in group of long-term cancer survivors who took our introductory eight-week program years ago. When we interviewed some of them about their experiences with meditation, they said that over time cancer became less and less a part of their identity. They ceased to be "cancer patients," "cancer victims," or even "cancer survivors" and just thought of themselves as people; meditators; or maybe writers, mothers, or whatever else occupied their energies, not defined primarily by their experience with cancer. This was a real relief to many of them; they were really tired of constantly thinking about cancer, reading about it, worrying that it might come back, and having it dominate their thoughts. Part of the healing process was this integration of the experience, moving beyond it and allowing other elements of who they were as developing human beings to emerge and flower.

HEALING OUR WORLD: MINDFULNESS IN COMMUNITY

Letting go of a narrow focus on the cancer experience and your personal worries allows you to develop greater awareness of others and their needs and desires. In fact, personal well-being and community well-being are interrelated and inextricably linked. The lyrics to the popular Jill Jackson Miller and Sy Miller song, *Let There Be Peace on Earth*—which essentially state that peace can and must begin within each of us—express this intuitive truth. Living mindfully offers the possibility of benefiting not only yourself and those close to you, but also your broader community.

How might that work? Sometimes people in our classes are so excited when they learn about mindfulness that they try to convince everyone around them to take up meditation and read this or that book. You can probably imagine the kind of reactions they get. Some people might be receptive, but the general response is often one of skepticism; they see it as the next trend someone's insisting they just *have* to try, probably another fad that will come and go in no time. People can sometimes take up the "cause" of mindfulness with a zealousness that tends to turn others off and elicit resistance or challenge.

We have found that the best way to promote mindfulness, if that's something you are inclined to do, is simply to be mindful in your everyday life. If you are committed and diligent, you can't fail to affect those around you. We routinely hear stories of spouses who remind each other to go and meditate when they've missed some sessions; they notice that their spouses are grouchier than when they are practicing. Truly practicing everyday mindfulness might include paying attention to the grocery clerk at the checkout, listening to what she says, and responding with kindness, rather than talking on your cell phone the whole time. It may mean not automatically yelling at your child for forgetting about homework for the umpteenth time, but rather listening to your child's explanation and responding with mindful consideration of the specific situation. That's not to say that this practice of remaining present with each unfolding moment of life is easy, but in our experience, no alternative offers greater gifts. Confining mindfulness to the meditation cushion doesn't really make much sense. Through formal practice, you build a solid foundation, but the wonder of a mindful life is the true fruit of practice.

The meditation in practice 14.2 is designed to strengthen the likelihood that you will remember to bring mindful awareness to your everyday interactions with others, and it can have a profound effect. It's similar to that concept of "pay it forward" where you purposefully do something kind or helpful for someone just because you can; in turn they are more likely to do the same for others. So in effect, you begin a cascade of goodwill by infusing your intentions and actions with a sincere concern for the well-being of not only yourself, but everyone else as well.

PRACTICE 14.2
Healing Meditation

Take a moment to find a comfortable seat where you can breathe easily and sustain an upright posture. As you begin to settle into the flowing rhythm of the breath, take a moment to check in with your body, mind, and spirit, noting how you find yourself today, accepting what you find without judging your thoughts or wishing things were different. Take a few minutes to allow the breath to settle and your focus to home in on the heart center, in the middle of your chest.

Now breathing in and out of the heart center, just noticing any sensations there—of warmth, expansion, or even nothing at all—accepting whatever's present—imagining drawing the breath down into this part of the body—as if breathing life into a small bubble that expands with each breath—while moving through the meditation, imagining this bubble filling with feelings of kindness and goodwill, and expanding breath by breath beyond the body and out into the world—while breathing out, sending a wish for healing and well-being, first to yourself—perhaps attaching a few phrases to each healing breath, such as May I be healed, May I be whole—*choosing from phrases of healing and kindness, such as* May I be well, May I share happiness—*continuing for several minutes.*

When the time is right, expanding this wish for healing beyond yourself to include others close to you in daily life—sending the wishes May you be healed, May you be whole, May you be free of conflict and struggle *to selected people in your life—noticing how it feels in your own body, in your heart center, to genuinely wish the best for others—recognizing that whatever their outward behavior, all people suffer, and like you, all people wish for happiness and healing in their lives—in recognition of this universal suffering, continuing to send out wishes for healing and peace—expanding beyond your own friends, family, and acquaintances to strangers, people you may pass in the street.*

Eventually, imagining the bubble of compassion in your heart expanding more and more to spread across the lands and oceans to people you may never meet in other parts of the world, people who are so in need of peace, healing, and reconciliation—repeating selected phrases with each inbreath and outbreath, such as May you be healed, May you be safe, May you be at peace.

After several more minutes of practice, when you are ready, opening your eyes and returning to the room, sensing the warm feeling you may have in your heart and body—seeing if you can carry that feeling with you into the world—extending healing, peace, and well-being to those you encounter in your daily life—recognizing that all beings suffer in ways you may not know, as well as other ways we have all experienced, and considering how you might turn this awareness into acts of kindness, compassion, or generosity that could benefit someone beyond yourself—despite their differing circumstances, recognizing and honoring in each person you encounter the same desire for health and happiness that you hold dear.

FINAL WORDS

We hope you have found this book useful and that it has supported you in discovering and aligning with your innate healing capacity. We included practical practices you can draw upon for years to come. We have also provided a reading list (see the appendix) including books and CDs we recommend for continued learning and practice in the areas of meditation, mindfulness, yoga, and mind-body medicine. We hope you continue to meet the world with your beginner's mind and discover new landscapes of possibility. We will do the same. Above all, may you be well, may you be happy, may you be whole, and may you be healed. In the words of one of our group participants:

> Cancer can make a person very bitter, or it can make them very wise. I'm not crazy about having had cancer, but it has certainly done a lot in my life.

APPENDIX

Reading List

MEDITATION INSTRUCTION

Books

Brantley, M., and T. Hanauer. 2008. *The Gift of Loving-Kindness: 100 Mindful Practices for Compassion, Generosity, and Forgiveness.* Oakland, CA: New Harbinger Publications.

Levey, J., and M. Levey. 1999. *Simple Meditation and Relaxation.* Berkeley, CA: Conari Press.

Levine, S. 1991. *Guided Meditations, Explorations, and Healings.* New York: Anchor Books.

Mipham, S. 2003. *Turning the Mind into an Ally.* New York: Riverhead Books.

Muller, W. 2000. *Sabbath: Finding Rest, Renewal, and Delight in Our Busy Lives.* New York: Bantam Books.

Smith, J. 1998. *Breath Sweeps Mind: A First Guide to Meditation Practice.* New York: Riverhead Books.

Yongey Mingyur Rinpoche. 2007. *The Joy of Living: Unlocking the Secret and Science of Happiness.* New York: Harmony Books.

Audio

Bodian, S. 2006. *Meditation for Dummies.* 2nd ed. Book and CD-ROM. Hoboken, NJ: Wiley Publishing.

Kabat-Zinn, J. 2002. *Guided Mindfulness Meditation.* Series 1. Four audio CDs. Stress Reduction CDs. www.mindfulnesscds.com.

———. 2002. *Guided Mindfulness Meditation.* Series 2. Four audio CDs. Stress Reduction CDs. www.mindfulnesscds.com.

———. 2005. *Guided Mindfulness Meditation.* Series 3. Four audio CDs. Saratoga Springs, NY: Galileo Multimedia. www.mindfulnesscds.com.

Salzberg, S., and J. Goldstein. 2002. *Insight Meditation.* Book and CD-ROM. Boulder, CO: Sounds True.

Weil, A., and J. Kabat-Zinn. 2001. *Meditation for Optimum Health: How to Use Mindfulness and Breathing to Heal Your Body and Refresh Your Mind.* Two audio CDs. Boulder, CO: Sounds True.

INSPIRATIONAL BOOKS ON MEDITATION

Kabat-Zinn, J. 1994; revised 2005. *Wherever You Go, There You Are: Mindfulness Meditation in Everyday Life.* New York: Hyperion.

Tolle, E. 1999. *The Power of Now: A Guide to Spiritual Enlightenment.* Novato, CA: New World Library.

———. 2003. *Stillness Speaks.* Novato, CA: New World Library; Vancouver, BC: Namaste Publishing.

MIND-BODY HEALTH

Borysenko, J. 2007. *Minding the Body, Mending the Mind.* With Larry Rothstein. Cambridge, MA: Da Capo Press.

Brantley, J. 2007. *Calming Your Anxious Mind: How Mindfulness and Compassion Can Free You from Anxiety, Fear, and Panic.* 2nd ed. Oakland, CA: New Harbinger Publications.

Davis, M., E. Robbins Eshelman, and M. McKay. 2008. *The Relaxation and Stress Reduction Workbook.* 6th ed. Oakland, CA: New Harbinger Publications.

Gardner-Nix, J. 2009. *The Mindfulness Solution to Pain: Step-by-Step Techniques for Chronic Pain Management.* With L. Costin-Hall. Oakland, CA: New Harbinger Publications.

Kabat-Zinn, J. 1990. *Full Catastrophe Living: Using the Wisdom of Your Body and Mind to Face Stress, Pain, and Illness.* New York: Delacorte Press.

———. 2005. *Coming to Our Senses: Healing Ourselves and the World Through Mindfulness.* New York: Hyperion.

Khalsa, D. S., and C. Stauth. 2002. *Meditation as Medicine: Activate the Power of Your Natural Healing Force.* New York: Fireside Books.

Martin, P. 1999. *The Healing Mind: The Vital Links Between Brain and Behavior, Immunity and Disease.* New York: St. Martin's Press.

Santorelli, S. 1999. *Heal Thy Self: Lessons on Mindfulness in Medicine.* New York: Bell Tower.

Thondup, T. 1998. *The Healing Power of the Mind: Simple Meditation Exercises for Health, Well-Being, and Enlightenment.* Boston: Shambhala Publications.

Williams, M., J. Teasdale, Z. Segal, and J. Kabat-Zinn. 2007. *The Mindful Way Through Depression: Freeing Yourself from Chronic Unhappiness.* New York: Guilford Press.

BUDDHIST

Bhante Henepola Gunaratana. 2002. *Mindfulness in Plain English*. Updated and expanded edition. Somerville, MA: Wisdom Publications.

Chodron, T. 2007. *Guided Meditation on the Stages of the Path*. Ithaca, NY: Snow Lion Publications.

Ferguson, G. 2009. *Natural Wakefulness: Discovering the Wisdom We Were Born With*. New York: Shambhala Publications.

Goldstein, J. 2003. *One Dharma: The Emerging Western Buddhism*. San Francisco: HarperSanFrancisco.

Kornfield, J. 1993. *A Path with Heart: A Guide Through the Perils and Promises of Spiritual Life*. New York: Bantam Books.

———. 2001. *After the Ecstasy, the Laundry: How the Heart Grows Wise on the Spiritual Path*. New York: Bantam Books.

Rosenberg, L. 1998. *Breath by Breath: The Liberating Practice of Insight Meditation*. With David Guy. Boston: Shambhala Publications.

Salzberg, S. 1995. *Lovingkindness: The Revolutionary Art of Happiness*. Boston: Shambhala Publications.

———. 1997. *A Heart as Wide as the World: Stories on the Path of Lovingkindness*. Boston: Shambhala Publications.

Thich Nhat Hanh. 1992. *Peace Is in Every Step: The Path of Mindfulness in Everyday Life*. New York: Bantam Books.

———. 2009. *You Are Here: Discovering the Magic of the Present Moment*. Boston: Shambhala Publications.

FAITH-GUIDED APPROACHES

Jewish

Lew, A. 2005. *Be Still and Get Going: A Jewish Meditation Practice for Real Life*. New York: Little, Brown, and Company.

Christian

Keating, T. 2006. *Open Mind, Open Heart: The Contemplative Dimension of the Gospel.* 20th anniversary ed. New York: Continuum International.

Merton, T. 2005. *No Man Is an Island.* Boston: Shambhala Publications.

Sufism

Azeemi, K. S. 2005. *Muraqaba: The Art and Science of Sufi Meditation.* Trans. S. S. Reaz. Houston, TX: Plato Publishing.

Rumi. 2004. *The Essential Rumi.* New expanded ed. Trans. C. Barks. With J. Moyne. San Francisco: HarperOne.

VISUALIZATION AND IMAGERY

Achterberg, J., B. Dossey, and L. Kolkmeier. 1994. *Rituals of Healing: Using Imagery for Health and Wellness.* New York: Bantam Books.

Naparstek, B. 1995. *Staying Well With Guided Imagery: How to Harness the Power of Your Imagination for Health and Healing.* New York: Warner Books.

Ornstein, R., and D. Sobel. 1999. *The Healing Brain: Breakthrough Discoveries About How the Brain Keeps Us Healthy.* Cambridge, MA: Malor Books.

YOGA AND STRETCHING

Books

Anderson, B. 2000. *Stretching.* 20th anniversary ed. Bolinas, CA: Shelter Publications.

Boccio, F. J. 2004. *Mindfulness Yoga: The Awakened Union of Breath, Body, and Mind.* Somerville, MA: Wisdom Publications.

Carrico, M. 1997. *Yoga Journal's Yoga Basics: The Essential Beginner's Guide to Yoga for a Lifetime of Health and Fitness.* New York: Henry Holt and Company.

Christensen, A. 1999. *American Yoga Association's Easy Does It Yoga: The Safe and Gentle Way to Health and Well-Being.* New York: Fireside.

Devi, N. J. 2000. *The Healing Path of Yoga: Time-Honored Wisdom and Scientifically Proven Methods that Alleviate Stress, Open Your Heart, and Enrich Your Life.* New York: Three Rivers Press.

Farhi, D. 1996. *The Breathing Book: Good Health and Vitality Through Essential Breath Work.* New York: Henry Holt and Company.

———. 2005. *Bringing Yoga to Life: The Everyday Practice of Enlightened Living.* San Francisco: HarperSanFrancisco.

Faulds, R. 2005. *Kripalu Yoga: A Guide to Practice On and Off the Mat.* New York: Bantam Books.

Feuerstein, G., and S. Bodian. 1993. *Living Yoga: A Comprehensive Guide for Daily Life.* New York: Putnam.

Holtby, L. 2004. *Healing Yoga for People Living with Cancer.* Lanham, MD: Taylor Trade Publishing.

Iyengar, B. K. S. 1995. *Light on Yoga.* Rev. ed. New York: Schocken Books.

Video

Grilley, P. 2005. *Yin Yoga: The Foundations of a Quiet Practice—With Paul Grilley.* DVD. San Francisco: Pranamaya. www.pranamaya.com.

Kabat-Zinn, J. 2010. *The World of Relaxation: A Guided Mindfulness Meditation Practice for Healing in the Hospital and/or at Home.* DVD. www.betterlisten.com.

Powers, S. 2005. *Insight Yoga with Sarah Powers.* Two DVDs. San Francisco: Pranamaya. www.pranamaya.com.

WEBSITES

Healing and Cancer is a Canadian website with varied resources for healing and cancer, at www.healingandcancer.org.

Anticancer is David Servan-Schreiber's website, based on his book *Anticancer: A New Way of Life*, at www.anticancerways.com.

Learning Meditation is a website featuring free, downloadable short audio and text meditations, at www.learningmeditation.com/room. htm.

References

Carey, M. P., and T. G. Burish. 1987. Providing relaxation training to cancer chemotherapy patients: A comparison of three delivery techniques. *Journal of Consulting and Clinical Psychology* 55 (5):732–37.

Carlson, L. E., and S. N. Garland. 2005. Impact of mindfulness-based stress reduction (MBSR) on sleep, mood, stress, and fatigue symptoms in cancer outpatients. *International Journal of Behavioral Medicine* 12 (4):278–85.

Carlson, L. E., M. Speca, P. Faris, and K. D. Patel. 2007. One-year pre-post intervention follow-up of psychological, immune, endocrine, and blood pressure outcomes of mindfulness-based stress reduction (MBSR) in breast and prostate cancer outpatients. *Brain, Behavior, and Immunity* 8:1038–49.

Carlson, L. E., M. Speca, K. D. Patel, and E. Goodey. 2003. Mindfulness-based stress reduction in relation to quality of life, mood, symptoms of stress, and immune parameters in breast and prostate cancer outpatients. *Psychosomatic Medicine* 65 (4):571–81.

———. 2004. Mindfulness-based stress reduction in relation to quality of life, mood, symptoms of stress and levels of cortisol, dehydroepiandrosterone sulfate (DHEAS), and melatonin in breast and prostate cancer outpatients. *Psychoneuroendocrinology* 29 (4):448–74.

Carlson, L. E., Z. Ursuliak, E. Goodey, M. Angen, and M. Speca. 2001. The effects of a mindfulness meditation–based stress reduction program on mood and symptoms of stress in cancer outpatients: Six-month follow-up. *Supportive Care in Cancer* 9 (2):112–23.

Cohen, S. 2005. Keynote presentation at the Eighth International Congress of Behavioral Medicine: The Pittsburgh common cold studies—Psychosocial predictors of susceptibility to respiratory infectious illness. *International Journal of Behavioral Medicine* 12 (3):123–31.

Feuerstein, G. 2000. *The Shambhala Encyclopedia of Yoga.* Boston: Shambhala Publications.

Garssen, B. 2004. Psychological factors and cancer development: Evidence after 30 years of research. *Clinical Psychology Review* 24 (3):315–38.

Greer, S., T. Morris, and K. W. Pettingale. 1979. Psychological response to breast cancer: Effect on outcome. *Lancet* 2 (8146):785–87.

Joyce, J. 2000 (1914). A painful case. In *Dubliners*, 103–14. London: Penguin.

Kabat-Zinn, J. 1990. *Full Catastrophe Living: Using the Wisdom of Your Body and Mind to Face Stress, Pain, and Illness.* New York: Delacorte Press.

Kabat-Zinn, J. 1994. *Wherever You Go, There You Are: Mindfulness Meditation in Everyday Life.* New York: Hyperion.

Kabat-Zinn, J., L. Lipworth, and R. Burney. 1985. The clinical use of mindfulness meditation for the self-regulation of chronic pain. *Journal of Behavioral Medicine* 8 (2):163–90.

Kabat-Zinn, J., L. Lipworth, R. Burney, and W. Sellers. 1986. Four-year follow-up of a meditation-based program for the self-regulation of chronic pain: Treatment outcomes and compliance. *Clinical Journal of Pain* 2 (3):159–73.

Mackenzie, M. J., L. E. Carlson, M. Munoz, and M. Speca. 2007. A qualitative study of self-perceived effects of mindfulness-based stress reduction (MBSR) in a psychosocial oncology setting. *Stress and Health* 23 (1):59–69.

Maunsell, E., J. Brisson, and L. Deschênes. 1995. Social support and survival among women with breast cancer. *Cancer* 76 (4):631–37.

Pearce, J. C. 1974. *Exploring the Crack in the Cosmic Egg: Split Minds and Meta-Realities.* 2nd ed. New York: Julian Press.

Salzberg, S. 2008. Metta: The practice of compassion. In *Quiet Mind: A Beginner's Guide to Meditation*, ed. S. Piver, 53. Boston: Shambhala Publications.

Savard, J., and C. M. Morin. 2001. Insomnia in the context of cancer: A review of a neglected problem. *Journal of Clinical Oncology* 19 (3):895–908.

Shapiro, Jr., D. H. 1992. Adverse effects of meditation: A preliminary investigation of long-term meditators. *International Journal of Psychosomatics* 39 (1–4):62–67.

Shapiro, S. L., L. E. Carlson, J. A. Astin, and B. Freedman. 2006. Mechanisms of mindfulness. *Journal of Clinical Psychology* 62 (3):373–86.

Sloman, R. 1995. Relaxation and the relief of cancer pain. *Nursing Clinics of North America* 30 (4):697–709.

Speca, M., L. E. Carlson, E. Goodey, and M. Angen. 2000. A randomized, wait-list controlled clinical trial: The effect of a mindfulness meditation–based stress reduction program on mood and symptoms of stress in cancer outpatients. *Psychosomatic Medicine* 62 (5):613–22.

Linda E. Carlson, Ph.D., R.Psych., holds the Enbridge Research Chair in Psychosocial Oncology, has won an Alberta Heritage Foundation for Medical Research Health Scholar award, and is associate professor in psychosocial oncology at the University of Calgary. She is director of psychosocial oncology research and works as a clinical psychologist at the Tom Baker Cancer Centre in Calgary, Canada. Carlson is coauthor of *The Art and Science of Mindfulness* and has published over ninety book chapters and research papers in peer-reviewed journals. She regularly presents her work at international conferences.

Michael Speca, Psy.D., R.Psych., is adjunct associate professor of psychosocial oncology at the University of Calgary and a former Canadian Cancer Society post-doctoral fellow at the Tom Baker Cancer Centre. As a clinical psychologist at the Centre, he counsels cancer patients and their families, facilitates a range of group support programs, and cofounded the Centre's popular Mindfulness-Based Cancer Recovery program.

Foreword writer Zindel Segal, Ph.D., is the Morgan Firestone Chair in Psychotherapy and professor of psychiatry at the University of Toronto. He is also director of the cognitive behavioral therapy unit at the Centre for Addiction and Mental Health and a founding fellow of the Academy of Cognitive Therapy. He is coauthor of *The Mindful Way Through Depression and Mindfulness-Based Cognitive Therapy for Depression.* He continues to advocate for the relevance of mindfulness-based clinical care in psychiatry and mental health.

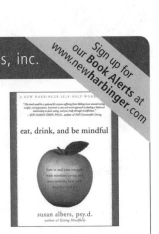
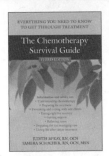
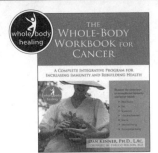
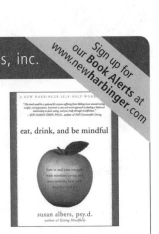
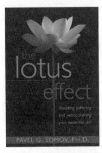
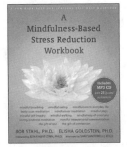
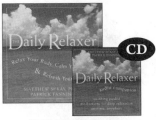